Handbook of Histology

Handbook of
Histology

KARL A. STILES, M.S., PH.D., SC.D.

Professor Emeritus of Zoology
Former Head of the Department of Zoology
Michigan State University

With an Introduction by
MELVIN H. KNISELY

Fifth Edition

The Blakiston Division
McGraw-Hill Book Company
New York   Toronto   Sydney   London

HANDBOOK OF HISTOLOGY

PREFACE

The enthusiastic reception and wide use of the four previous editions of this handbook demonstrate that it has been a valuable "road map" in histology for the beginning student. It is a supplementary textbook of histology with considerable emphasis on the diagnostic characteristics of tissues and organs. The fifth edition is based on the same general plan as the others but with improvements such as the inclusion of ultrastructure of the common cell as seen with the electron microscope. New illustrations have been included, new summary charts have been added, and parts of the text have been thoroughly revised. The glossary has been enlarged and pronunciation included, and the bibliography has been expanded. This new edition reflects the valuable suggestions of many instructors and students who have been using the handbook.

There is a tendency for textbooks of histology to become so voluminous that they take on the character of reference books. The beginning student scans such a book with a feeling of discouragement and futility, under the impression that he will be expected to remember all the histologic minutiae which it contains. Only as the course progresses does he begin to realize that much of the subject matter is for reference, but even then he has great difficulty in distinguishing the grain from the chaff, a task for which he is poorly equipped. This handbook attempts to separate one from the other; it assists the student of histology in the organization of his information and helps him to simplify the mastery of this very important discipline. Because it is not a reference book, controversial topics have been largely omitted. Where controversial material is unavoidable, the dominant concepts have been adopted. Many graphic tables make large accumulations of knowledge easier to learn.

Diagrammatic line drawings of the fundamental tissues have been used because most teachers prefer them to high-power photomicrographs, since the drawings can be made to include several focal planes.

This handbook can be used as a laboratory manual. Since the premedical or medical student of histology has had some microscopic anatomy, detailed laboratory directions are unnecessary. It may be used as a syllabus with lectures. Some teachers use the handbook in their classes as a basis for review. It has also proved its worth for purposes of review to students of pathology. Students preparing for "spot" quizzes and for state and national board examinations find it invaluable. This volume is also useful in preparation for the many specialty boards requiring a review of the basic sciences. Regardless of the method of handling histology instruction, this book will be very helpful in guiding the student in identification studies of tissues and organs in the laboratory.

Blank pages have been included for lecture or laboratory notes and drawings. In fact, many instructors require their students to make laboratory drawings in the handbook, thus making it more valuable for reference purposes. Some students have requested more illustrations, but histology instructors in general are of the opinion that the handbook is of greater value to the student if he furnishes his own illustrations made from actual preparations studied in the laboratory.

Color illustrations have their place in a textbook of histology, but the author feels that for this kind of supplementary text, the cost is difficult to justify. Furthermore, many teachers have found that students using colored illustrations tend to identify tissues by color rather than structure, which is deplorable.

KARL A. STILES

ACKNOWLEDGMENTS

The author desires to express his appreciation to the students and instructors who offered advice and suggestions during the preparation of this revised text. He wishes especially to acknowledge his indebtedness to Dr. Robert Burns, Kenyon College, Gambier, Ohio; Drs. A. W. Stimson, M. L. Calhoun, and Esther M. Smith, Department of Anatomy, Michigan State University; Dr. Paul A. Walker, Biology Dept., Randolph-Macon Woman's College; Dr. L. M. Ashley, Walla Walla College; Dr. R. A. Runnells, Department of Animal Pathology, Michigan State University; Dr. R. A. Fennel, Department of Zoology, Michigan State University; Estelle Downer, Milwaukee County General Hospital; Bernadette McCarthy Henderson, Department of Zoology, Michigan State University; Dr. G. E. Braunschneider, Grand Rapids, Michigan; Dr. John E. Luke, East Lansing, Mich., Dr. R. Dean Schick, State Teachers College, Cortland, N.Y., Dr. Douglas Eastwood, University of Iowa, and Particia A. Harris, Boston, Mass. Special thanks go to the author's wife, Nettie R. Stiles, who spent many hours in the preparation and proofreading of this handbook.

K.A.S.

CONTENTS

PREFACE   *v*

ACKNOWLEDGMENTS   *vii*

INTRODUCTION   *xiii*

LIST OF TABLES   *xi*

1. How to Interpret Sections   1
2. How to Identify Tissues and Organs   6
3. Cell Structure and Division   10
4. Epithelial Tissues   22
5. Connective Tissues   36
6. Reticuloendothelial (Macrophage) System   54
7. Human Blood and Lymph   58
8. Muscular Tissue   66
9. Nervous Tissue   72
10. The Circulatory System   86
11. Lymphatic (Lymphoid) Organs   102
12. Skin and Its Appendages   112
13. Digestive System   122
14. Glands of the Digestive System   148
15. Respiratory System   154
16. Urinary System   162
17. Male Reproductive System   170
18. Female Reproductive System   180
19. Endocrine System   194
20. Eye   204
21. Ear   212
22. Olfactory Organ   218
23. Taste (Gustatory) Organ   220
24. Tissues and Organs Sometimes Confused   221
25. Summary of Main Distribution of Cartilage   223
    Glossary   225
    Selected References   241
    Index   243

TABLES

1. Classification of Simple Epithelial Tissues with Their Embryonic Origin and Location 28
2. Classification of Stratified Epithelial Tissues with Their Embyronic Origin and Location 29
3. Summary of the Formed Elements of Human Blood 64
4. Special Features of the Three Types of Muscles, as an Aid to Diagnosis 70
5. Summary of the Histology of the Circulatory System . . . 98–100
6. Summary of the Histology of the Lymphatic Organs 110
7. Summary of the Histology of the Digestive System 144–147
8. Summary of the Histology of the Respiratory System 160–161
9. Summary of the Histology of the Urinary System 168–169
10. Summary of the Histology of the Male Reproductive System . 178–179
11. Summary of the Histology of the Female Reproductive System . . 192

INTRODUCTION

Histologic studies are made for a definite purpose: to collect evidence for the development of accurate concepts of the structure, function, and response of the small parts of normal living bodies. With accurate information on the structure and behavior of small parts, we can deal inductively with these facts and understand the functions of whole organs and systems.

Each animal lives in four dimensions, three of space and one of time. At any moment, each feature of an animal's anatomy exists in the three space dimensions. But many features of the spatial architecture undergo rapid or slow cyclic, intermittent, or progressive changes with time. The chemical and physical characteristics, the shapes, the magnitudes, and the positions of structure change as parts of development, of physiology, and of pathology. New structures appear and old ones disappear. These are changes along the time dimension.

A histologic section is only part of the original living animal; it is a two-dimensional slice out of a four-dimensional system, minus what has been lost, plus that which has been added in its preservation and preparation for study. From serial sections we mentally construct some concepts of the three dimensions of living structures. To gain concepts of the changes of structure with time, a group of animals are selected and all are treated alike in the hope they will respond alike in direction, degree, and rate. After certain time intervals, a few are selected, from each of which two-dimensional sections are made. From the resulting static pictures, and by constructive imagination, mental concepts of life processes are synthesized.

A course in histology has at least two major purposes: (1) to help the student understand the structure and function of living things and (2) to give the student mental pictures of the two-dimension slices of "normal" organs. These picture concepts of normal organs serve as a model against which to recognize and judge the abnormality of obviously altered organs. Each of these major purposes demands that the student be able to recognize as many dead tissues as possible and that he have firmly in mind the salient characteristics of each tissue and organ. For developing concepts of living microscopic anatomy, it is just as important for the histologist to know the structure of tissues and organs as it is for a mathematician to know the multiplication table or the relationships commonly expressed in elementary algebra. The great complexity cannot be dealt with at all without a firm foundation, which in this case is the precise knowledge of the structure of sections of dead tissues and organs.

In too many courses in histology a large part of the time is spent teaching students to recognize histologic sections of tissues and organs. It is deplorable that students should have to waste so much time on this necessary but elementary phase of the subject. Would a mathematics department have its students spend a corresponding proportion of time on the multiplication table?

The important functions of this book are to help students learn to recognize tissues rapidly and to fix firmly in their minds the descriptive phrases which go with the salient features of the microscope image pictures presented by histologic sections. The handbook is a necessity, it presents outlines of the subject matter, it separates the trees from the forest; had Dr. Stiles not written the book, others would have attempted it. The book has great value to the student and teacher because it assists in rapid learning of a group of basic phrase-plus-picture concepts, which is one of the necessary first steps toward learning and understanding the microscopic structure and functionings of living tissues and organs.

MELVIN H. KNISELY
Professor and Chairman of the Department of Anatomy
Medical College of South Carolina
Charleston, South Carolina

Chapter 1

HOW TO INTERPRET SECTIONS

Histology is the study of microscopic anatomy. The earliest histologists were of necessity restricted to the unaided eye and simple lenses in their observations of tissues and organs. The improvement of the microscope and the development of new techniques with modern optical instruments have made possible great advances in the study of tissues. Most histology today is learned from the study of sections, thin slices cut through the various tissues and organs.

Slices cut through different planes or at various levels of an organ may give diverse impressions about its structure. As is shown in Fig. 1, no single slice of a hard-boiled egg gives a correct idea of its structure. To obtain the whole picture of the structure of a complicated organ, it is necessary to study several sections taken from different sites and in different planes. This also demonstrates why a given section of an organ may not look the same under the microscope as it does in a textbook illustration.

When one looks at a section, he should try to visualize how it was cut. The student will gain help in doing this if he forms a mental image of some familiar object cut at different angles. Most of the organs of the vertebrate animal body contain tubes, partitions, and cords; and examples of these are, respectively, blood vessels, septa (partitions of connective tissue) in the spleen, and nerve cords. If the student knows how straight tubes, partitions, and bundles of cords appear in slices cut at different angles (Figs. 2, 3, and 4), he will not only gain skill in recognizing these structures, but he will also be able to better visualize similar structures of the body when they are cut in different planes.

It is, therefore, very helpful in interpreting sections to become familiar with the appearances of slices of straight tubes, partitions, and cords. Figures 2, 3, and 4 should give such assistance with this problem. The student will save a great deal of time if he studies these carefully, and then, as he undertakes the study of histologic sections, refers back to these figures frequently. Finally, he should try to visualize the structure of the entire tissue or organ from a series of sections. This involves making mental reconstructions in three dimensions when only two are actually seen.

1

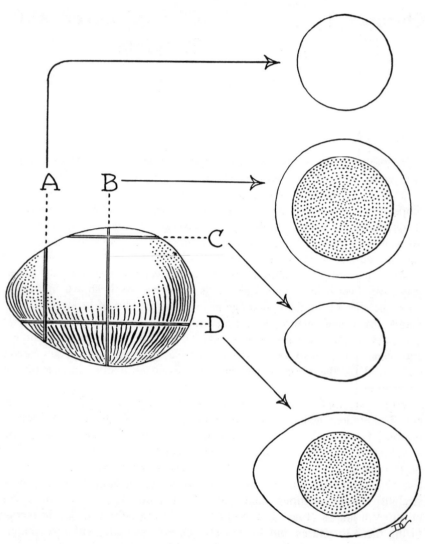

Fig. 1. Diagrams showing how sections cut through an object at different levels or in different planes may give different ideas regarding its structure. (Courtesy of A. W. Ham, Histology, 2d ed., J. B. Lippincott Company, Philadelphia, 1953.)

Thin slices cut through a straight tube as at the left of this figure appear <u>as below</u> when mounted on glass slides.

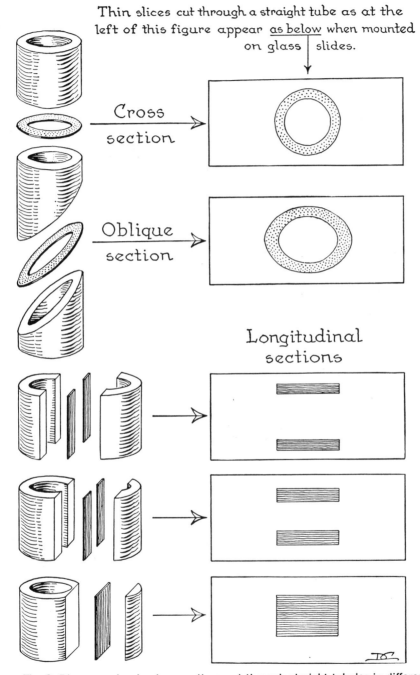

Cross section

Oblique section

Longitudinal sections

Fig. 2. Diagrams showing how sections cut through straight tubules in different planes appear different when mounted on a slide and observed through the microscope. Note that it is possible to cut a longitudinal section of a tube without the lumen showing in the section. (Courtesy of A. W. Ham, Histology, 2d ed., J. B. Lippincott Company, Philadelphia, 1953.)

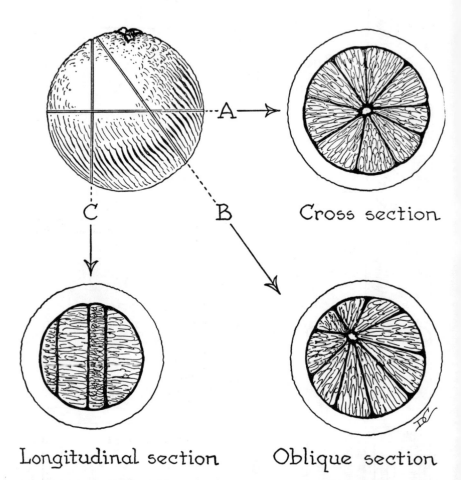

Cross section

Longitudinal section   Oblique section

Fig. 3. Diagrams showing the different appearances presented by sections cut in different planes through an object which contains partitions (an orange). (Courtesy of A. W. Ham, Histology, 2d ed., J. B. Lippincott Company, Philadelphia, 1953.)

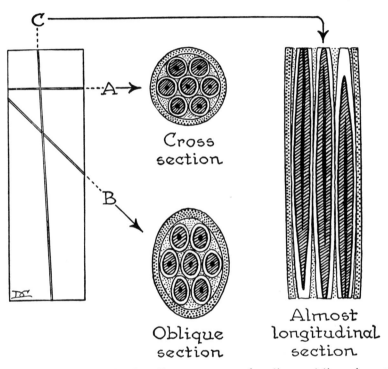

Cross
section

Oblique
section

Almost
longitudinal
section

Fig. 4. Diagrams showing how the appearance of sections cut through a cable containing many insulated wires differs according to the plane in which the section is cut. (Courtesy of A. W. Ham, Histology, 2d ed., J. B. Lippincott Company, Philadelphia, 1953.)

Chapter 2

HOW TO IDENTIFY TISSUES AND ORGANS

In commencing a laboratory study of histology, it is difficult to select from the confusing abundance of histologic information that which is most helpful for the purpose of recognizing tissues. This handbook should help the beginning student to overcome this difficulty.

An outline of this sort, however, has certain limitations. While only the principal characteristics of tissues and organs have been included, with some emphasis on identification characters, it cannot be too strongly emphasized that the more complete the information one has about an organ the better he is prepared for an accurate diagnosis of a complex of tissues.

The beginning student in histology is likely to fall into the error of considering one good "spotting" character for a tissue sufficient, but this is erroneous; identification work is not that simple. It should be remembered that tissues are subject to the variations which occur in all living things, and constant exceptions will be found to almost any generalization. Also, the possibility must be considered that in any given section a favorite identifying character may be absent. For example, the pancreas may be identified positively by the presence of the islands of Langerhans; but if a section does not possess islands, then the tissue may be easily confused with parotid, unless one is fortified with a complete knowledge of the histology of the organ. Then, too, the histology of organs varies in different animals, depending on how far the animals are removed from one another phylogenetically. Despite the desirability of knowing as much as possible about the histologic structure of the organ to be identified, *the author has acceded to a general student demand that some of the most diagnostic characters be italicized.*

For the benefit of medical students who look forward to work in pathology, it may be said that certain tissues and organs show profound changes under the influence of disease. For instance, in fatty atrophy of the pancreas, only islands of Langerhans may be present; or, in voluntary muscle, only the neuromuscular spindles may persist. One who knows the neuromuscular spindles will recognize the area in which one is found as a region of striated muscle even though no contractile fiber is present. Under the influence of postmortem changes, only the stroma of organs may persist. Thus, the spleen can be recognized by the persistence of the characteristic trabeculae even though no stainable nuclei remain to identify the splenic pulp cells. In pathology it is necessary to know the diagnostic characteristics which are most likely to persist when the organ is seriously altered by disease.

The descriptions given here are based largely on the tissues of man and other higher vertebrates; and, unless otherwise specified, the stain referred to is hematoxylin and eosin.

METHODS OF MICROSCOPIC IDENTIFICATION OF TISSUES AND ORGANS

Tissues and organs are recognized in two ways: (1) *by superficial recognition of tissues, the picture made by the tissue as a whole; (2) by recognition of elements: the tissue elements are first identified, then a deduction is made as to the tissue's identity.*

The Superficial Recognition Method

This is a poor method, and too often used by the beginning student of histology. It depends entirely on visual memory of the general pattern made by the tissues of a structure; the tissue is identified as parotid gland because it looks like it. This method is likely to fail if there is something about the histologic picture which makes it appear unfamiliar. Unfamiliarity may be due to three causes: (1) the inclusion of structures not normally present; (2) the exclusion of parts usually present; and (3) the presentation of familiar parts in a new way. Thus a tissue may be readily recognized when stained with hematoxylin and eosin, but if stained with only iron hematoxylin it may be very difficult to identify because of the difference in color pattern.

While a student may be able to identify correctly 95 percent of the histologic preparations in a set of slides which he has studied, he may be able to identify only 50 percent in an identification test with other slides. The difference between these two scores results from the student having learned to diagnose his own histologic preparations by purely superficial means; he identifies tissues by color, shape of section, or something else besides the form and arrangement of tissue elements. A good way to test one's dependence on superficial characters is to place a piece of colored cellophane in the blue glass carrier underneath the condenser of the microscope. This changes the color of the preparation. The difficulty now encountered in identification is in direct ratio to the superficial methods which have previously been used. Another way to overcome the tendency to make superficial identifications is to write out a list of the structures observed in a preparation before making a histologic diagnosis.

The Recognition-of-elements Method

This method, which is employed by histologists, is as follows:

1. Look at the preparation with either the naked eye or with a reversed ocular to see whether it is composed of one or more types of tissue. Often some general idea may be gained as to the size and shape of the parts of certain organs.

2. Examine the section under a low-power (32-mm) objective, using a low-power eyepiece. Identify as many of the different kinds of tissues as possible. Then note carefully the relationship of the various tissues to one another. Many organs can be identified with such an examination, but they should also be examined with a higher power for confirmation of diagnosis. Since most medical microscopes are not equipped with a 32-mm objective, it may be necessary to omit this step.

3. Examine the section under a 16-mm objective, using a low-power (10×) eyepiece. If possible, study the cellular character of the tissue. Often the cellular structure is not distinct, yet much may be told about the general cellular nature from the position and relation of the nuclei to one another.

Methodically examine the cells in different parts of the specimen. Classify them according to the relative area occupied by cells and by matrix. If the matrix is small in amount, the cells are probably epithelial or glandular. If the cells are surrounded by much matrix, connective tissue is indicated. It may sometimes be found desirable to use a higher power than a 16-mm objective and a 10× ocular for a detailed study of cells, but this is rarely the case.

4. Keep the different classes of fundamental tissues in mind, and mentally visualize the arrangement of the different tissues of the preparation under consideration.

The various regions of the body where such tissues could occur in close apposition should now be considered. Each of such tissues or organs has certain special features, and the specimen should now be examined for the presence of these special features. *By a process of elimination of the impossible, identity of the tissue or organ is determined.* Failure to identify a satisfactory preparation by this method will mean that the student does not know the fundamental tissues or that he has an inadequate knowledge of special histology (microscopic structure of organs). Do not base an identification on a single field since the region may be atypical due to artifacts or pathologic changes.

In the electron microscope, the light source used in the light microscope is replaced by electrons emitted by a tungsten filament; magnetic or electric fields take the place of the glass lenses; and a fluorescent screen is used for viewing. The requirements for using an electron microscope, and the special treatment and preparation of tissues, result in a highly complex and expensive system.

However, the electron microscope has shown that the cell is much more complicated in structure than has heretofore been thought. The most striking developments in the structure of the cell are pointed out in this handbook, so that the student may be aware of what is happening in the field of microscopy, even though it is not practical for the individual student to use an electron microscope.

Chapter 3

CELL STRUCTURE AND DIVISION

Cells are the biologic building stones of all tissues. Most cells consist of a small mass of protoplasm, which consists of cytoplasm and a nucleus enclosed by a membrane. The cell is the structural, functional, hereditary, and developmental unit of an organism. In its functions the cell can assimilate, grow, reproduce, and respond to external stimuli.

CELL STRUCTURE

A. Cytoplasm

This constitutes the protoplasm of a cell exclusive of the nucleus. It is usually bound externally by a *cell membrane* (*plasma membrane, plasmalemma*). Within the cytoplasm are numerous bodies which may be divided into two separate categories as follows (Fig. 5):

1. **ORGANELLES (ORGANOIDS).** These bodies are differentiated parts of the cytoplasm. They are permanent parts of a cell and act like "cell organs."

   a. CENTROSOME (CELL CENTER). When present it lies near the nucleus. The centrosome consists of a sphere of clear cytoplasm, the *centrosphere*, in which lie one or two dark-staining granules, the *centrioles*, referred to collectively as the *diplosome*. The centrioles are readily demonstrated with iron hematoxylin. By electron microscopy, a centriole is a rodlike structure containing nine sets of peripheral rodlets and two sets of central rodlets. Some authors use the term *centrosome* synonymously with *centriole*.

   b. MITOCHONDRIA. These can be demonstrated in living cells with dark-field and phase-contrast microscope techniques. They vary in shape from granules to long filaments. Some stain supravitally with Janus green. By electron microscopy, mitochondria are membranous structures consisting of an outer smooth membrane and an inner limiting membrane with cristae continuous with the inner limiting membrane (Fig. 5).

ULTRASTRUCTURE OF THE COMMON
CELL ORGANELLES AND INCLUSIONS

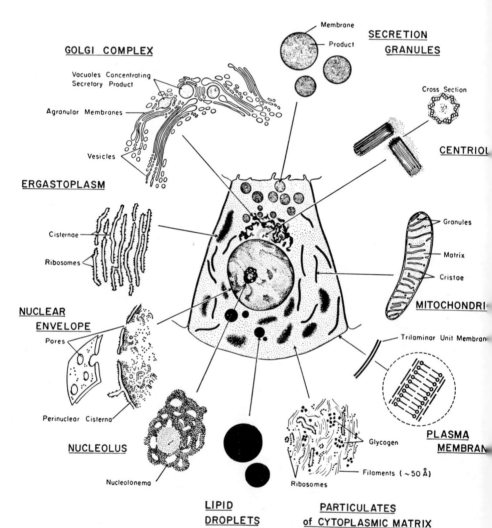

Fig. 5. In the center of this figure is a diagram of the cell illustrating the form of its organelles and inclusions as they appear by light microscopy. Around the periphery are representations of the finer structure of these same components as seen in electron micrographs. The ergastoplasm of light microscopy consists of aggregations of submicroscopic membrane-limited elements with granules of ribonucleoprotein adhering to their outer surface. These elements constitute what is now also called the granular or rough endoplasmic reticulum. The illustration of the plasma membrane encircled by an interrupted line does not show structure that has been directly observed but represents one possible interpretation of the arrangement of lipid and protein molecules that may be related to the trilaminar appearance of cell membranes in electron micrographs. (Courtesy of William Bloom and Don W. Fawcett, A Textbook of Histology, 8th ed., W. B. Saunders Company, Philadelphia, 1964.)

c. GOLGI APPARATUS. The Golgi apparatus varies considerably from one cell to another, even in the same cell, depending on the functional stage. It is described in some cases as a dense network of fibrils; in other cases, as stacked piles of flat protein-filled sacs. In electron micrographs the Golgi apparatus consists of parallel arrays of membranes and numerous small vesicles (Fig. 5). The smooth-surfaced membranes of the Golgi apparatus are continuous with the rough-surfaced membranes of the endoplasmic reticulum.

(1) Secretions. The Golgi apparatus is secretory in function. It is involved in the import and export of materials and seems to serve as a site for materials produced in other parts of the cells. The substance in the Golgi apparatus is principally phospholipid. The Golgi apparatus shows acid and alkaline phosphatase activity, and that of other enzymes.

d. ENDOPLASMIC RETICULUM AND ERGASTOPLASM. The cytoplasmic membranes continuous with the plasma membrane and the outer nuclear membrane constitute the endoplasmic reticulum. The ergastoplasm includes that part of the endoplasmic reticulum which has two characteristics: (1) networks of canaliculi, flattened sacs, and vacuoles that have a limiting membrane and (2) dense granules of ribonucleoprotein (RNP, ribosomes) spaced along the outer surface of the membranes. The endoplasmic reticulum associated with ribosomes is usually called the rough-surfaced (granular) endoplasmic reticulum (Fig. 5). *The ribonucleoprotein fraction of the cell is the site of protein synthesis,* and there is good evidence that the lamellar portion of the endoplasmic reticulum synthesizes cholesterol and other sterols. The smooth-surfaced endoplasmic reticulum is called the agranular endoplasmic reticulum; it does not have the granules of ribonucleoprotein. A specialized form of the smooth-surfaced endoplasmic reticulum is the Golgi apparatus. It has been shown that there are communications between the rough-surfaced and smooth-surfaced endoplasmic reticulum.

e. FIBRILS (FIBRILLAE). Definite fibrils may be observed in muscle cells, nerve cells, macrophages, epithelial cells, and many other types of cells. The ultrastructure shows that a fibril consists of lamellae. The fibril is not now regarded as a part of the fundamental structure of all cytoplasm.

f. LYSOSOMES. Above the mitochondria in centrifuged specimens is a fluffy layer of particles called lysosomes, which contain hydrolytic enzymes. The internal structure of lysosomes varies in appearance under the electron beam. Lysosomes are sur-

rounded by a limiting membrane that isolates the enzymes from the remainder of the cell. It is thought that lysosomes provide the enzymes for digestion of some of the materials taken into the cells.

2. **CYTOPLASMIC INCLUSIONS.** Cytoplasmic inclusions comprise accumulations of material which are not constant. Whether all materials in this category are nonliving is a matter open to question (Fig. 5).

   a. SECRETION GRANULES AND GLOBULES

   b. STORED FOODS. Carbohydrates, fats, and proteins.

   c. PIGMENTS. Colored granules occur in some cells. Melanin is the most common pigment.

3. **CELL MEMBRANE (PLASMA MEMBRANE, PLASMALEMMA)**

The cell membrane is the structural boundary between the cytoplasm and that which surrounds the cell (Fig. 5). Its physical and chemical abilities control passage of materials in and out of the cell, a property known as permeability. The cell membrane contains:

   a. MICROVILLI. These are numerous folds in the surface of the cell. A cell may have 3,000 of these.

     (1) Brush Border. The microvilli of renal tubular epithelium vary greatly in length, some branching, thus forming an enormous absorptive surface, which is called a brush border.

     (2) Striated Border. The microvilli of the intestinal epithelium are of the same length and are independent of each other, and appear as a striated border.

     (3) Stereocilia. The stereocilia in the ductus epididymis are branching surface modifications. They are actually microvilli and not cilia because they do not have the characteristic filament structure and motility of cilia.

     (4) Cilia and Flagella. Cilia are a motile form of the specialization of the surface of the cell. Cilia are short and numerous; flagella are long and few in number.

     (5) Desmosomes. Electron microscopy shows points of mechanical attachment between cells called desmosomes. They are found in the juxtaluminal portion of the cell. They are dense discontinuous thickenings of apposing plasma membranes. Fine filaments converge onto the desmosomes from the cell cytoplasm.

     (6) Terminal Bars. These are closer to the lumen than desmosomes. They are local specializations of the surfaces of adjacent cells that maintain a firmer attachment to other cells.

(7) Intercellular Bridges. These are not open communications between cells as it was once believed, but are sites of end-to-end contact of short processes on adjacent cells. At the points of contact the cells are firmly attached by surface specializations called desmosomes.

(8) Interdigitation of Cell Surfaces. In cells closely associated, the plasma membrane of the cells may show complex in-infolding and dovetailing. This increases the surface of the plasma membrane and may facilitate transport of material into or out of cells (as in salivary duct or renal tubular epithelium) or accommodate expansion of a cavity (as in urinary bladder epithelium).

B. Nucleus

The nucleus is usually a spherical, ovoid, or elliptical body. It is delimited from the cytoplasm by a nuclear membrane. By electron microscopy, the nuclear membrane is a double membranous envelope (Fig. 5).

1. DIFFERENTIATED SUBSTANCES OF THE NUCLEOPLASM

a. NUCLEAR SAP. A fluid ground substance which fills the nucleus.

b. NUCLEOLUS. The nucleolus is typically a small spherical body; it may contain one or more nucleoli. It cannot be seen during some stages of mitosis.

c. CHROMOSOMES. These are Feulgen-positive bodies of characteristic shape and size, which are most conspicuous during cell division. A discussion of the minute structure of the chromosome is beyond the scope of this book.

CELL DIVISION

Reproduction, growth, and repair of tissues depend on some form of cell multiplication. Cells are reproduced by a process of division.

A. Amitosis (Direct Cell Division)

This is considered a rare method of cell division. It is generally thought to occur only in pathologic, senescent, and certain highly specialized transient tissues such as erythrocytes and placental cells.

1. IN AMITOSIS the nucleus of an *interphase* (*"resting"*) *cell* merely constricts near the middle and finally separates into two portions. Fission of the cytoplasm may follow soon after the divi-

sion of the nucleus. True examples of amitosis are rare. Whether amitosis actually exists at all is controversial.

B. Mitosis (Indirect Cell Division)

The reproduction of most cells involves a series of nuclear processes of considerable complexity. Four stages are usually described:

1. **PROPHASE.** This stage is characterized by a series of changes through which the very fine threads of the interphase cell nucleus are changed in form to the thicker and more conspicuous chromosomes of the metaphase. The nucleolus and nuclear membrane disappear in this stage.
   a. Simultaneously with the development of the chromosomes, the centrioles move to opposite sides of the nucleus.
   b. The formation of rays around each centriole results in the development of a structure known as the aster.
   c. Threads form which reach from the chromosomes to the asters. These threads are called spindle fibers.
   d. Threads that reach from one aster to the other are termed continuous spindle fibers.

2. **METAPHASE.** In the interphase preceding the prophase, a "split" of chromosome occurs; apparently each chromosome reproduces an exact copy of itself, thus duplicating deoxyribonucleic acid (DNA), the genetic material. Later the "split" chromosomes separate farther. The diagnostic feature in the metaphase is that the chromosomes become located in the equatorial plane of the mitotic figure.

3. **ANAPHASE.** This is the period in which the two sets of chromosomes resulting from longitudinal "splitting," move to opposite poles of the cell.

4. **TELOPHASE.** The two groups of chromosomes now in the vicinity of the asters are reconstructed into the nuclei of typical interphase cells. A division of the cytoplasm takes place to form the daughter cells. The nucleolus which disappeared during the process of mitosis is reformed, and the spindle fibers gradually disappear.

C. Meiosis

This is a form of cell division restricted to gametes or germ cells. It has as its major functions the reduction of chromosomes by half (from the diploid to the haploid number) and the production of genetic variation.

Chapter 4 EPITHELIAL TISSUES

The functions of the epithelium are sensory reception, protection, secretion, excretion, lubrication, absorption, and reproduction.

The epithelial tissues described in this chapter are those having one surface bordering a space or a cavity and a second surface usually adjoining an underlying basement membrane. This latter structure is often so thin as to be imperceptible in routine preparations.

Epithelial cells may also be arranged in the form of solid cords or masses, e.g., parathyroids; in the form of follicles, e.g., thyroid glands; or in indefinite arrangements, e.g., thymus; but these will be considered in subsequent chapters under the histology of organs.

In the epithelial tissues *only a small amount of intercellular substance is present. Cell borders are usually indistinct, and it is difficult to determine where one cell ends and another begins.* Cells are arranged in a single layer (simple) or in several layers (stratified). Identification is based largely on the shape of the cells in profile view (Fig. 6*B*). The free surfaces of the cells may be ciliated (Fig. 6*F*) or nonciliated (Fig. 6*H*).

Epithelial sheets on the body surface are avascular; that is, blood vessels do not penetrate among the epithelial cells.

Protoplasmic interconnections known as intercellular bridges are usually described as occurring in epithelia in general. Yet they are most conspicuous in the lower layers of stratified epithelia.

A. Simple (Single-layered) Epithelia[1]

1. **SQUAMOUS.** *Examples:* nonciliated—tympanic cavity; posterior epithelium of the cornea; lining of blood vessels and heart (endothelium); lining of peritoneal, pleural, and pericardial cavities (mesothelium); and portions of uriniferous tubules and rete testes.

Although endothelium and mesothelium are unquestionably morphologically epithelium, some pathologists prefer to consider them apart from the ordinary epithelium because the cells behave differently from other epithelial cells in repair of inflammations

---

[1] Some teachers prefer to have students study columnar epithelium first because it is easier to study.

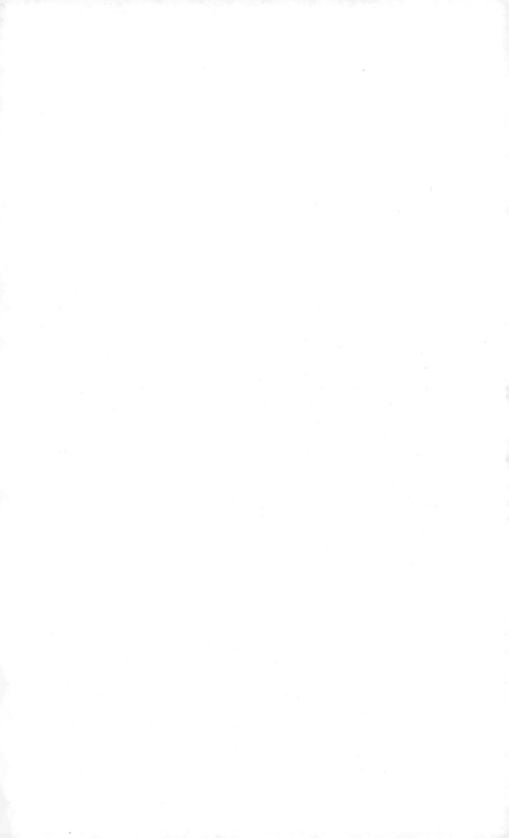

and in tumor growth. Inasmuch as the classification adopted for this book is primarily morphologic, we include endothelium and mesothelium under the heading of epithelium.

   a. In profile view, *cells appear as thin plates of protoplasm, their midportion, where the nucleus is located, forming a prominent bulge on the free surface* (Fig. 6*B*).

   b. Usually with one free flat surface (Fig. 6*A*).

2. **CUBOIDAL.** *Examples:* nonciliated—thyroid follicular cells and kidney tubules; ciliated—mouse uterus.

   a. Nuclei are approximately equidistant from cell membranes.

   b. In vertical section the cells appear to be nearly square (Fig. 6*D*).

3. **COLUMNAR.** *Examples:* nonciliated—intestine; ciliated—oviduct (Fig. 6*E*).

   a. Tall prismatic cells, *whose basal nuclei in vertical sections are crowded and are all practically at the same level.* Compare with cuboidal (Fig. 6*D*).

   b. Striated (striped) border with terminal bars. *Example:* intestine.

4. **PSEUDOSTRATIFIED.** *Examples:* nonciliated—male urethra and excretory duct of parotid; ciliated—trachea and large bronchi.

   a. *Two to four layers of nuclei which give a stratified appearance* (Fig. 6*F*).

   b. *Nuclei occupy approximately two-thirds of the epithelial layer.* Compare with stratified columnar epithelium.

   c. Surface cells are columnar and always touch the relatively thick basement membrane of the epithelial sheet. Basal cells which are not columnar do not extend to the free surface. Thus in a pseudostratified epithelium, all cells touch the basement membrane but not all reach the surface.

   d. Usually ciliated.

   e. Vertical sections of pseudostratified epithelium and tangential sections of simple columnar epithelium are easily confused. However, in pseudostratified the nuclei are of several types, those at the base of the tissue are small and dark, those nearer the surface, larger and paler. In the tangential section of columnar epithelium, although nuclei may appear at different levels, they are all of one type.

B. Stratified (Many-layered) Epithelia

These are characterized by two or more layers of cells (Fig. 6*G*). *The kind of stratified epithelium is determined by the shape of the cells in the outer layer or free surface.*

1. **SQUAMOUS.** *Examples:* cornea, part of the conjunctiva, epidermis of skin, mouth, esophagus, vagina, and part of the female urethra.
   a. *Surface cells usually flat or scalelike.* They differ from the cells of simple squamous epithelium in that they possess *flat nuclei* which do not produce an enlargement of the cell.
   b. *Often with papillated lower border.*
   c. Sometimes a transition from basophilic to acidophilic staining capacity from the base of the epithelial sheet to its surface.
   d. *Basal nuclear layer pronounced.*
   e. Cell membranes may be distinct or indistinct.
   f. Arrangement:
      (1) Deepest cells are soft and delicate—one layer.
      (2) Intermediate cells are polygonal in outline, larger. Intercellular bridges of cytoplasm bind them together.
      (3) Superficial layers are flattened by pressure.
   g. *Examples:*
      (1) Corneal Epithelium
         (a) Four to six layers of cells, nonpapillated.
         (b) *Only stratified squamous epithelium without connective tissue papillae.*
      (2) Skin Epithelium
         (a) Tall papillae of connective tissue penetrate the epithelial layer. Considered in the order from without inward the layers are corneum, lucidum, granulosum, and germinativum.
         (b) Thin skin shows only the stratum germinativum and stratum corneum clearly.

2. **TRANSITIONAL.** *Examples:* pelvis of kidney, ureter, urinary bladder (Fig. 6*I*), and prostate portion of male urethra. This epithelium is limited in distribution to the urinary tract.
   a. The cells at the free surface of transitional epithelium are described by some authors as pear- or balloon-shaped, but by others as somewhat flattened or broadly cuboidal. Actually the same section may show both balloon-shaped and broad cuboidal cells next to the lumen. This condition appears to be due to the fact that the broad cuboidal cells at the free surface rest on a layer of balloon-shaped cells, and that there is considerable desquamation of the surface cells, *leaving the balloon- or dome-shaped cells at the free margin* in certain areas. The frequency with which the superficial cells are found in urine is an indication of the extent to which desquamation of these cells takes place.
   b. *Concave facets on the under surface of the surface cells are diagnostic in clinical examinations of urine.*

    c. Surface cells are thicker than superficial scaly cells of stratified squamous epithelium.

    d. *Nuclei of surface cells tend to be more spherical than in stratified squamous epithelium.* This description applies to relaxed transitional epithelium. When this epithelium is stretched the cells become much flattened (Fig. 6*J*).

    e. Relatively smaller number of cell layers than in stratified squamous epithelium. *Transitional, usually not more than three to ten cells deep.*

TABLE 1. CLASSIFICATION OF SIMPLE EPITHELIAL TISSUES WITH THEIR EMBRYONIC ORIGIN AND LOCATION

Kind	Ectoderm	Mesoderm	Entoderm
Squamous: Nonciliated	Membranous labyrinth, amnion, and chorion	Endothelium and mesothelium, posterior epithelium of cornea, rete testis, Henle's loop of kidney	Tympanic cavity, mastoid cells
Cuboidal: Nonciliated	Anterior surface of lens, covering of iris and ciliary body, choroid plexus, pigmented epithelium of retina, membranous labyrinth (external spiral sulcus)	Follicular cells of ovary, collecting tubules of kidney	Smallest bronchioles, small bile ducts, small pancreatic ducts, thyroid follicular cells
Ciliated		Part of uriniferous tubule in the mouse	
Columnar: Nonciliated	Organ of Corti, taste buds, ducts of salivary glands	Part of collecting ducts of kidney	Alimentary canal (stomach to anus), gallbladder
Ciliated	Embryonic ependyma of brain and of cord	Uterus, oviduct	Bronchioles
Pseudostratified: Nonciliated		Part of ductus deferens	
Ciliated	Respiratory part of nasal cavity		Trachea, bronchi, part of larynx, eustachian tube

TABLE 2. CLASSIFICATION OF STRATIFIED EPITHELIAL TISSUES WITH THEIR EMBRYONIC ORIGIN AND LOCATION

Kind	Ectoderm	Mesoderm	Entoderm
Squamous: Nonciliated	Epidermis, lips, ocular conjunctiva, anal canal, oral cavity, external nares, external auditory tubes, tear ducts, fossa navicularis of urethra, vulva	Vagina, part of cervix	Pharynx, esophagus, part of larynx, vocal cords, part of epiglottis
Columnar: Nonciliated	Palpebral conjunctiva, cavernous urethra, olfactory membrane	Part of ductus deferens	Part of larynx
Transitional: Nonciliated		Pelvis of kidney, ureter, part of urinary bladder	Part of urinary bladder, part of urethra

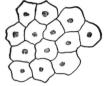

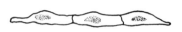

A. SIMPLE SQUAMOUS—Surface view   *B.* SIMPLE SQUAMOUS—Profile

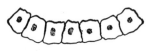

C. CUBOIDAL OR COLUMNAR—Surface view   *D.* SIMPLE CUBOIDAL—Profile

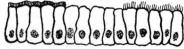

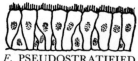

E. SIMPLE COLUMNAR—Profile
(Left side with striated border, right side ciliated)

F. PSEUDOSTRATIFIED
(Ciliated)

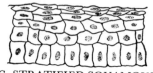

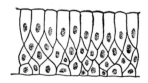

G. STRATIFIED SQUAMOUS
(Noncornified)

H. STRATIFIED COLUMNAR
(Nonciliated)

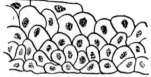

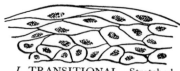

I. TRANSITIONAL—Collapsed
(Showing two types of surface cells)

J. TRANSITIONAL—Stretched

Fig. 6. Diagrams of types of epithelium. Each tissue is shown in vertical section unless described otherwise.

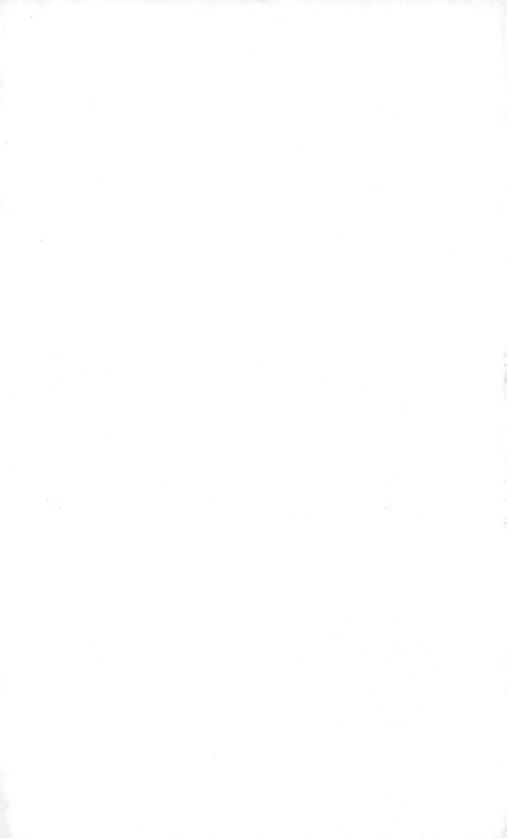

f. Practically no formation of keratin (horny material) in transitional epithelium.

g. *Nonpapillated,* hence basal line usually more regular.

3. COLUMNAR. *Example:* part of pharynx.

a. Relatively rare type of epithelium (Fig. *6H*).

b. *Outer cells always columnar; inner cells may appear cuboidal.*

c. *Nuclear portion comprises three-fourths to four-fifths of the entire epithelial layer.* Compare with pseudostratified epithelium.

d. Numerous nuclei, compact and ovoid.

e. Basal nuclei form a more nearly straight row as contrasted with the irregular arrangement in pseudostratified epithelium.

f. Goblet cells may or may not be present.

g. Mucosa not papillated.

NOTE: See Tables 1 and 2, pp. 28 and 29, and Fig. 7, p. 32, for summaries on epithelial tissues.

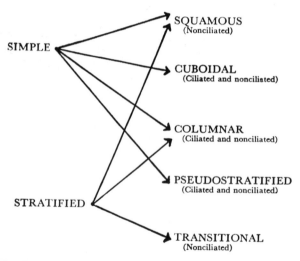

Fig. 7. Diagram summarizing the types of epithelial tissues.

C. Glandular Epithelia

1. UNICELLULAR GLANDS

a. GOBLET CELLS. *Example:* intestine, especially colon.

2. MULTICELLULAR GLANDS

a. MUCOUS CELLS. *Examples:* sublingual and submaxillary glands, surface layer of the stomach and uterus.

   (1) Large triangular cells with nuclei sometimes flattened and near basement membrane. Alveoli with small but definite lumen.

(2) *Cytoplasm, staining poorly with hematoxylin, is pale slate blue or colorless.*

  b. SEROUS (ALBUMINOUS) CELLS. *Example:* parotid gland.

    (1) Smaller than mucous cells. Slightly eccentric spherical nucleus, although it varies with secretory cycle. Practically no visible lumen in alveoli.

    (2) *Cytoplasm granular* and more or less basophilic. Appearance differs with secretory cycle. Basal striations may be present.

  c. SEROMUCOUS (MIXED) GLANDS. *Examples:* submaxillary and sublingual glands. Because they contain both mucous and serous cells these are known as seromucous (mixed) glands.

    (1) The intrinsic part of the mixed alveolus usually consists of mucous cells. But attached to the alveolus, at the point farthest away from the intercalated duct, is a thin biconcave cap of serous cells. These cells form the crescent of Giannuzzi (demilunes).

  d. GLANDS NEITHER MUCOUS NOR SEROUS. *Examples:* liver and kidney. They do not constitute a group that is united by similarities of structure or function. They are mentioned here merely to point out that many glands exist which cannot be classified as either serous or mucous. Because they are so varied they will be discussed individually in later chapters.

D. Pigmented Epithelia. *Examples:* external epithelium of retina, ciliary body, and to some degree the basal layer of the stratum germinativum.

1. Cells contain large quantities of pigment granules.

E. Neuroepithelia. *Examples:* taste buds of tongue and auditory sense cells. Various localized sensory regions in epithelium consisting of cells of special types not represented in the taste buds or auditory sense cells.

Chapter 5   CONNECTIVE TISSUES

The connective tissues are the supporting or uniting structures of the body.

Connective tissues are characterized primarily by the paucity of cells and the dominance of variable amounts and numerous types of substances, such as fluid, mucus, and fibers.

Most connective tissues originate from the same type of mesodermal tissue, and mesenchyme. But a special condition is found both in the nervous system, where the supporting tissue, the neuroglia, is in part derived from the ectoderm, and in the thymus, where the reticulum is derived from the entoderm.

Connective tissue is classified into several types which represent specializations of structure for various special functions. However, classification is difficult as various types of adult tissues are not sharply separated from one another, so any attempt to place these tissues in many distinct categories is certain to be artificial; therefore the classification below is quite general.

I. EMBRYONIC CONNECTIVE TISSUE

A. Mesenchyme (Mesenchyma). *Example:* in early embryo, packing material between the external and internal epithelial layers (Fig. 8*A*).

1. Consists of loosely arranged cells with slender branching processes which appear to be continuous from one cell to another, forming a network. Recent studies suggest that mesenchyme is composed of discrete cells and that the processes are merely adherent to neighboring cells.
2. In fixed preparations the cytoplasm is scanty; a large nucleus appears to occupy most of the cell.
3. The cell membranes are indistinct.
4. Spaces between the cells are filled with a semifluid substance in living tissue.

NOTE: The terminology of this primitive type of connective tissue

is not well standardized. Therefore some authors use the term *mesenchyme* synonymously with *embryonal* or *mucous;* others use the terms *embryonic* and *embryonal* synonymously; and still others use *mesenchyme* and *embryonic* synonymously. This multiplicity of terminology is likely to prove confusing to a beginning student of histology, and this statement is made in the hope that it will help resolve the difficulty.

B. Mucous Tissue. *Examples:* Wharton's jelly of the umbilical cord and vitreous humor of the eye.

1. Intercellular spaces filled with a jellylike mucoid substance.
2. Nuclei, oval or elongated, to conform with the shape of the cell.
3. Borders of the stellate or spindle-shaped cells are indistinct.
4. *A few eosinophilic collagenous fibers.*
5. Some of the fibers are single, while others unite to form wavy bundles.
6. *Example:* umbilical cord (Fig. 8*B*).
   a. Periphery covered with flattened epithelial cells.
   b. Intercellular spaces filled with large amount of mucous substance, Wharton's jelly.
   c. Interior may show one vein and two arteries with much muscle in the vessel walls.
   d. The older the cord is, the larger the cross section; and with more fibers occurring, fewer cells are present.
   e. If the section is taken from a part of the cord near the body of the embryo, the yolk sac may be present. This may prove very confusing to a beginning histologist.

II. ADULT CONNECTIVE TISSUE

A. General

1. **LOOSE (AREOLAR) CONNECTIVE TISSUE.** *Example:* superficial fascia (Fig. 8*G*).
   a. Collagenous (white) fibers, elastic fibers, a few reticular fibers. Bundles of fibers which are cut transversely, obliquely, and longitudinally are intermingled in cross section.
   b. With hematoxylin and eosin stain, it may be difficult to distinguish between elastic and white fibers, but with the electron microscope, collagenous connective tissue fibers have a highly characteristic and distinctive cross-striation. Collagen is the principal fibrous protein of connective tissue and appears as wavy, ribbonlike bands that stain with acid dyes. With the elec-

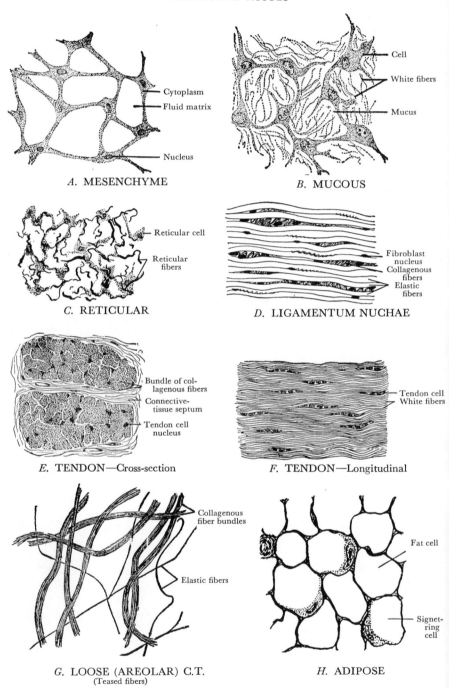

A. MESENCHYME

B. MUCOUS

C. RETICULAR

D. LIGAMENTUM NUCHAE

E. TENDON—Cross-section

F. TENDON—Longitudinal

G. LOOSE (AREOLAR) C.T.
(Teased fibers)

H. ADIPOSE

Fig. 8. Diagrams of types of connective tissue.

tron microscope they appear as aggregates of small fibers. It is believed that collagen is formed extracellularly by the growing of a prefibrillar protein, which is completed by the cell, usually a fibroblast.

c. *No definite arrangement of fibers.*

d. Types of cells: fibroblasts, mesenchymal cells, macrophages (histiocytes), chromatophores, leucocytes, eosinophils, plasma cells, fat cells, and a small number of mast cells.

e. An amorphous ground substance in which fibers and cells are embedded.

2. **DENSE CONNECTIVE TISSUE.** *Examples:* in the dermis of the skin, the submucous layer of the intestine, and parts of the urinary tract.

a. PARALLEL FIBERS (REGULAR). These are more or less regularly arranged to withstand tension exerted in one direction.

(1) Predominantly Collagenous. *Examples:* tendons and ligaments. These fibers are closely packed, parallel, and frequently wavy; nuclei between fiber bundles.
A cross-section (Fig. 8E) may show tendon cells (fibroblasts) irregular in shape with cytoplasmic processes extending from main bodies. Ligaments are similar to tendons except that the elements are less regularly arranged. Some are composed almost entirely of elastic fibers.

(2) Predominantly Elastic. These fibers are less numerous than the closely packed collagenous type. *Examples:* vocal cords and ligamentum nuchae.

b. INTERLACED FIBERS (IRREGULAR). Close packing of fibers. A feltlike structure, constructed to withstand tensions exerted from different directions.

(1) Predominantly Collagenous. *Examples:* dermis of skin, deep fascia, capsules of organs (spleen, testis); sheaths (periosteum of bone); septa and trabeculae (partitions within organs); and perichondrium.

(2) Predominantly Elastic. *Example:* within blood vessels.

B. Special Tissues

1. **RETICULAR TISSUE.** *Examples:* framework of bone marrow, liver, lymph nodes, spleen, thymus, and other lymphoid tissues (Fig. 8C).

a. Characterized by a cellular reticulum as well as *argyrophilic fibers which branch and anastomose to form diffuse networks.* These fibers may be clearly demonstrated with silver nitrate. The details of the reticular cells, however, cannot be observed in such preparations.

b. *The spaces of the reticular network are filled for the most part with lymph and lymphocytes,* but this is not so in bone marrow, liver, and endocrine organs.

c. Reticular cells may be in close relation to the fibers of the reticulum. By electron microscopy they may be observed to lie upon and, in some instances, surround the fibers.

2. **ELASTIC (YELLOW) TISSUE.** *Example:* ligamentum flava of the vertebrae and fenestrated membrane of the larger arteries.

a. Living fibers are yellow in color and elastic in the common sense of the word.

b. *Each fiber appears to be a structureless homogeneous thread.*

c. Fibers branch and anastomose.

d. *Example:* ligamentum nuchae (Fig. 8D), often used for demonstration purposes in student laboratories because of the enormous size of the fibers, but for this same reason it is atypical of elastic fibers.

   (1) Large eosinophilic fibers that curl at the ends.

   (2) *Fibers are dense,* running mainly in one direction.

   (3) *No nuclei in fibers, but nuclei between fibers rather than between fiber bundles as in tendon.*

3. **ADIPOSE TISSUE.** *Examples:* outer part of capsule of kidney, in the omentum, and in adult mesentery. *It is peculiar because its bulk consists of cells instead of intercellular substance.*

a. *Signet-ring cells may be present,* i.e., cells with the nucleus pushed to one side of the cell membrane (Fig. 8H).

b. *Cells appear vacuolated because the intracellular fat substance is removed in preparation* (Fig. 8H).

c. *Nuclei not observed in every cell,* because fat cells are so large and histologic sections so thin that fat-cell nuclei may not be included in a section.

d. Groups of cells separated by loose connective tissue.

4. **PIGMENTED TISSUE.** *Examples:* choroid of the eye and lamina fusca of the sclera of the eye. These are described in the chapter on the eye.

a. The majority of the cells in the loose connective tissue are pigment cells (melanophores); therefore it has been called "pigment tissue."

C. Cartilage (Gristle)

1. **PRECARTILAGE.** *Example:* embryonic digit (Fig. 9A).

a. No matrix, or matrix reduced to a minimum.

b. Cells small and very numerous.

2. **HYALINE CARTILAGE.** *Example:* tracheal rings (Fig. 9*B*).
   a. *Like ground glass in appearance,* with basophilic matrix. Although no specific fibers are ordinarily seen, yet the matrix is permeated by a felt-like structure of fine collagenous fibrils.
   b. Each cell is enclosed within a *small space* (*lacuna*) which it completely fills during life. In mature cartilage there may be as many as four cells in a lacuna. Cells with prominent nuclei and clear cytoplasm.
   c. Much more matrix than in precartilage.
   d. Covered by perichondrium except over the articular surfaces of bone.

3. **ELASTIC CARTILAGE.** *Examples:* external ear, Eustachian tube, epiglottis, and in some of the laryngeal cartilages (Fig. 9*E*).
   a. *Similar to hyaline cartilage, plus a large number of branching yellow fibers between the lacunae.*
   b. Staining of intercellular substance surrounding the capsule is dense compared with hyaline cartilage.
   c. Often distinctly eosinophilic.
   d. Capsules[1] and cells more or less prominent.
   e. Cells likely to form in smaller groups than in hyaline cartilage.

4. **WHITE FIBROCARTILAGE (FIBROUS CARTILAGE).** *Examples:* intervertebral disk (Fig. 9*D*) and junction of tendon and bone.
   a. Differs in appearance from dense white fibrous tissue, such as ligaments and tendons, in that *the meshes of the dense fibrous tissue are permeated by cartilage cells.*
   b. *The cells are usually widely separated and arranged in rows, but differ from tendon cells in their ovoid shape and in the presence of cartilage capsules,* although these are not well differentiated.
   c. Immediate pericapsular territories are usually free from collagenous fibers.
   d. *The fiber bundles, which are slightly eosinophilic, run a wavy course through the matrix.* Fibers usually run parallel with one another.
   e. Plates of fibrocartilage are not surrounded by a perichondrium.

5. **ARTICULAR CARTILAGE.** *Example:* covering of the articular surfaces of the bones (Fig. 9*C*).
   a. *Usually hyaline cartilage without perichondrium, and with cells*

---

[1] The walls of lacunae of adult cartilage are more highly refractive than the surrounding matrix; they stain intensely with basic dyes, and are said to form capsules.

CONNECTIVE TISSUES

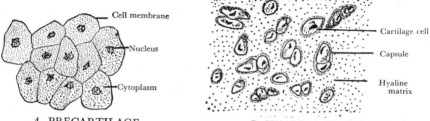

A. PRECARTILAGE

B. HYALINE CARTILAGE

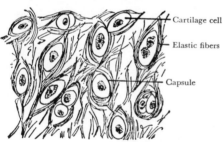

C. ARTICULAR CARTILAGE

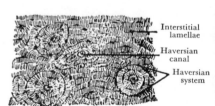

D. WHITE FIBROCARTILAGE

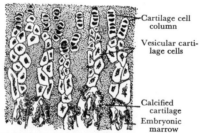

E. ELASTIC CARTILAGE

F. COMPACT BONE

G. DEVELOPING INTRACARTILAGINOUS BONE

Fig. 9. Diagrams of types of connective tissue.

near one surface greatly flattened. Other cartilage cells in short columnar groups.
b. Cancellous bone usually found on one side.

D. Bone

The difference between spongy (cancellous) bone and compact bone is a matter of architecture rather than histology. Fundamentally the composition of the bone matrix, its lamellation, and the relations of the bone cells to the matrix are the same in both cases. It is the way in which the bone matrix is arranged that distinguishes one type of bone from the other. Spongy bone is composed of a lattice work of slender trabeculae enclosing large numbers of marrow spaces. In compact bone there is a secondary deposit of lamellae in the marrow spaces, thus increasing the density of the bone as a whole.

1. **SPONGY (CANCELLOUS).** *Examples:* flat bones of skull and in the epiphysis of long bones.
   a. Irregular trabeculae of bone with bone cells, but *without Haversian canals.*
   b. Blood cells and red bone marrow in the marrow spaces between the trabeculae.
   c. Young bone usually shows edge of trabeculae beaded with osteoblasts.

2. **COMPACT.** *Example:* diaphysis of long bone in cross section.
   a. *Haversian canals surrounded by concentric lamellae of bone* (Fig. 9F). Haversian canals are channels running longitudinally in the substance of the bone and containing blood vessels, lymphatics, nerves, and Volkmann's canals.
   b. Interstitial lamellae between Haversian lamellae.
   c. Lacunae distinct with canaliculi.
   d. Canaliculi, tiny canals, extend from one lacuna to another.
   e. Stains pink in decalcified and bluish in calcified sections.
   f. Periosteum of connective tissue.

E. Development of Bone (Osteogenesis)

1. **INTRAMEMBRANOUS OSSIFICATION.** *Examples:* bones of the vault of the cranium and flat bones of face and jaw (membrane bones).
   a. Osteoblasts are formed directly from mesenchymal cells. Among the transforming mesenchymal cells appear collagenous fibrils. Between the cells and fibrils is an interstitial matrix; both the fibrillar element and the interstitial matrix are elaborated by

the cell. When mineralization of the bone occurs, a formless substance clouds the matrix and apatite crystals form. Apatite crystals develop both in and on the collagenous fibers. Further crystallization apparently occurs spontaneously.

b. Osteoblasts become entrapped within the matrix to form osteocytes of mature bone.

2. **INTRACARTILAGINOUS (ENDOCHONDRAL) OSSIFICATION.** *Example:* Inner portion of a long bone (Fig. 9G).

a. Preexisting cartilage is replaced by bone, hence this is sometimes called cartilage replacement bone. Cartilage degeneration is followed by bone formation.

b. The essential process of intracartilaginous bone formation is like that which occurs in intramembranous bone.

Chapter 6   RETICULOENDOTHELIAL (MACROPHAGE) SYSTEM

The *reticuloendothelial system* is a collective term applied to *all the phagocytes of the body except the leukocytes.* Besides clearing the blood stream of particulate matter, they are also engaged in lipoid metabolism and in the breakdown of hemoglobin. These phagocytes are derived from the mesenchyme, and are believed capable of forming blood cells and fibroblasts when the body is under great stress. Thus the system is very important in the economy and defense of the body.

Unfortunately, the cells of this system are not distinguished by any single morphologic characteristic. For study purposes, they are best identified by their marked ability to engulf particulate matter which has been intravenously injected with stains such as trypan blue, lithium carmine, or India ink (vital staining). Silver stains are also of value in observing the reticulum of certain organs. Cells of this system are found in every organ of the body, and vary in appearance according to their location.

A. Macrophages (Histiocytes, Resting Wandering Cells, Clasmatocytes)

1. Occur in loose connective tissue such as subcutaneous tissue and fascia.
2. Cells irregular in outline with short blunt processes.
3. *Resemble fibroblasts, but nuclei are smaller and denser.*
4. Cytoplasm coarsely granular.

B. Kupffer Cells (Stellate Cells of Kupffer)

1. Found only in the liver; they are interspersed with the endothelial cells lining the liver sinusoids.
2. Cells stellate in outline; numerous processes.
3. *Kupffer cells are distinctly larger than those of the accompanying endothelium.*

C. Reticular Cells of Lymphoid Tissue

1. Reticular cells and their fibers form the meshlike framework of lymphoid organs and aggregations. In lymph nodes, they are also interspersed with the endothelial cells lining the lymph sinuses; in the spleen they have a comparable position in blood sinuses.
2. Thin cytoplasmic extensions touch those of other cells.
3. *Nuclei stain lightly.*

D. Reticular Cells of Red Bone Marrow

1. Form a meshlike framework, as in lymphoid organs.
2. Resemble the reticular cells of lymphoid tissue.

E. Microglia

1. Occur only in nervous tissue.
   a. More numerous in gray matter than in white.
   b. Frequently found close to the cell bodies of neurons.
   c. Often in contact with blood vessels.
2. Nucleus small, dense, usually irregular in outline; *resembles the fibroblast nucleus.*
3. Cytoplasm scant; slender processes invisible without special stains.

F. Others

1. Lining cells of the sinusoids of the adrenal gland and hypophysis (pituitary gland).
2. Free macrophages found in the alveoli of the lungs. Large cells with pale cytoplasm. When they contain particles of dust, they are called "dust cells." There is some question about including these cells as a part of the reticuloendothelial system for they do not phagocytose vital stains, and, what is more important, there is the possibility that they are not of mesenchymal origin.

Chapter 7   HUMAN BLOOD AND LYMPH

Blood may be considered one type of atypical connective tissue, consisting of free cells (corpuscles) and a fluid intercellular substance (plasma). The mesenchyme of mesodermal origin gives rise to the blood as well as to most of the connective tissues. Thus it is evident that blood is both structurally and genetically related to connective tissue. Functionally, however, it does not fit into the connective tissue picture, for connective tissue is usually defined as a medium of support, or connection between the various body structures.

A. Red Blood Corpuscles (Erythrocytes, Erythroplastids)

1. These are recognized by their pink color,[1] *dark borders, and light central areas which do not contain nuclei.*
2. They are the most numerous of the formed elements in the blood.
   Male, about 5,500,000 per cu mm.
   Female, about 5,000,000 per cu mm.
   Average approximately 8.5 microns in diameter. In a given section, the erythrocytes furnish a useful gauge for estimating the size of other structures.

3. **CRENATED CORPUSCLES**
   a. These are shrunken erythrocytes (ghosts) on the surface of which are spine or knoblike processes.

4. **ROULEAU**
   a. Refers to the tendency of erythrocytes to become arranged like coins in a pile.

B. White Corpuscles (Leukocytes)

1. These are true cells for they contain nuclei. Some granules may be found in the cytoplasm of the lymphocytes and monocytes, but the granules in the polymorphonuclear cells are usually more distinct

---

[1] All colors of blood corpuscles refer to preparations stained with Wright's blood stain.

and in great abundance. About 5,000 to 9,000 cells per cu mm
Size of cell varies with type.

a. Agranulocytes (cytoplasm without granules, or with azurophilic granules).

   (1) Lymphocytes

      (a) Cells are small, medium, and large, the small being
most common. They are larger than erythrocytes, with
a relatively large nucleus, about which there may be a
narrow rim of slightly basophilic cytoplasm. *In some
the cytoplasm is so scanty that only the large spherical
nucleus is distinguishable.* The nucleus of large lymphocytes may be located at one side of the cell. Percentage: 20–25%.[1] Size: 7–10 microns.

   (2) Monocytes (large mononuclear leukocytes)

      (a) Cells which are typically larger than lymphocytes,
though they cannot always be sharply differentiated
from some of the larger lymphocytes. *The typical
monocyte has far more cytoplasm than a lymphocyte;
and the nucleus, usually eccentric in position, is
round, oval, slightly indented, or crescent in shape.*
The chromatin is finer, the nucleus is paler than that
of a lymphocyte, and the cytoplasm is faintly basophilic with occasional granules. Percentage: 3–8%.
Size: 12–15 microns.

b. Granulocytes (cytoplasm contains specific granules, that is,
either neutrophilic, eosinophilic, or basophilic granules). The
granules by electron microscopy are membrane-bounded granules of complex structure. They contain hydrolytic enzymes active at acid pH and are of the class of lysosomes.

   (1) Polymorphonuclear Leukocytes. These are so named because the nucleus is lobed. These blood cells are generally
larger than erythrocytes.

      (a) Neutrophils (heterophils)

         (*1*) Cells almost twice the size of an erythrocyte. *The
nucleus is highly polymorphous. May be elongated
with a bent or twisted body which consists of
several irregular, thin, nuclear threads.* The number of lobes varies from two to five, the most
common number being three. Percentages based
on character of nucleus: 5–12% band-form
nuclei (stab cells); 50–60%, two to five lobes;

---

[1] All percentages relative to the blood refer to the total number of leukocytes
in man.

and 3%, more than five lobes. The cytoplasm is
finely granular and stains a faint lilac to salmon
pink in color. Percentage: 58–75%. Size:
9–12 microns.

(b) Eosinophils (acidophils).

(1) Cells about twice the size of an erythrocyte. *The
nucleus often has two oval lobes connected by a
nuclear thread. The cytoplasm contains coarse
refractive granules which stain a red color.* Percentage: 2–5%. Size: 10–14 microns.

(c) Basophils.

(1) Cells which are somewhat larger than an erythrocyte. *The nucleus is usually bent in the form of
an S and is provided with two or more constrictions. It is usually centrally placed and stains
faintly. The cytoplasm contains very large irregular granules which stain a deep blue color.* These
coarse granules often completely obscure the nucleus. Percentage: 0.5–1%. Size: 8–10 microns.

NOTE: The diameters given for the leukocytes refer to living blood.
The size in smears is quite variable, but in general, a cell is larger in
smear preparation, due to stretching and flattening.

C. Blood Platelets (Thrombocytes, Thromboplastids)

1. Platelets are fragments of cytoplasm, important in the clotting of
blood. In fresh blood, stained and dried on a slide, they appear
singly, but more often in clumps. The clear, slightly blue cytoplasm
(called hyalomere) is usually filled with azurophilic granules.

D. Blood Plasma

1. Plasma is 55% of blood, while cellular elements constitute 45%.
2. The plasma appears most often as a granular, but structureless,
mass. The fibrous elements (fibrin) appear as fine to coarse interlacing threads.

E. Lymph

1. Composition.
   a. A liquid collected by the lymphatic vessels from all over the
   body. In the thoracic duct it contains a large number of cells.
   About 99% of these cells are lymphocytes. There may be a
   few erythrocytes, an occasional eosinophilic leukocyte, but
   rarely a monocyte.

TABLE 3. SUMMARY OF THE FORMED ELEMENTS OF HUMAN BLOOD

Type of Cell	Diameter, Microns	Nucleus	Cytoplasmic Granules Wright's Stain	Numbers or Percentages per Cubic Millimeter	Phagocytic Properties
Erythrocytes	About 7.5	None	None	Male, about 5,500,000; female, about 5,000,000	Absent
Lymphocytes	7–10	Spherical	About 10% with azuro-philic granulation	20–25%	Slightly phagocytic
Monocytes (Mononuclear leukocytes)	12–15	Usually eccentric in position. Round, oval, slightly indented, or crescentic in shape	Usually fine azurophilic granulation	3–8%	Highly phagocytic; engulf particulate matter
Neutrophils (Heterophils)	9–12	Highly polymorphous. Elongated, bent, or twisted body, with two to five lobes connected by thin nuclear threads	Neutrophilic. Stain faint lilac to salmon-pink color	60–75%	Highly phagocytic; ingest small, discrete particles as cinnabar, carbon, and bacteria
Eosinophils	10–14	Usually two oval lobes connected by a chromatic thread	Coarse, refractive. Stain red	2–5%	Phagocytic
Basophils	8–10	Usually bent in the form of S; provided with two or more constrictions	Large, irregular. Stain deep blue	0.5–1%	Phagocytic
Blood Platelets	About 3	None	Azurophilic	Average about 200,000 to 300,000	Absent

Leukocytes

64

Chapter 8   MUSCULAR TISSUE

A. Smooth Muscle (Nonstriated or Involuntary Muscle). *Examples:* gastrointestinal muscle, muscle of urinary bladder, and uterine muscle.

1. LONGITUDINAL SECTION

    a. Cytoplasm of the muscle fiber exhibits vague longitudinal markings which in special preparations prove to be longitudinal myofibrils (myofibrillae).

    b. *A single central elongated nucleus within each cell,* but the nucleus may be coiled when the cell is contracted.

    c. In many structures in which smooth muscle occurs, the cells (fibers) are close together and form a more or less definite muscular membrane in which the outlines of the cells may not be distinguishable. *May be confused with connective tissue, from which it is distinguished by the position of the nuclei which are within the fibers.*

    d. No distinct sarcolemma present, but by electron microscopy a condensed extracellular ground substance similar in some respects to basement membrane may surround a smooth muscle cell and contribute to the appearance of sarcolemma as seen in the light microscope.

    e. With hematoxylin and eosin, smooth muscle stains more darkly than connective tissue fibers and is not so refractive.

2. CROSS SECTION

    a. *The position of the nucleus is in the central portion of the cells.*

    b. *The difference in size and form of cells occurring in the same bundle is due to the fact that the fusiform cells may be cut through the thick central portion or at the narrow ends.*

    c. Cells covered by so thin a membrane that it is imperceptible in ordinary preparations.

    d. *Smooth muscle is less eosinophilic than striated voluntary muscle or cardiac muscle.*

B. Skeletal Muscle[1] (Striated Muscle). (Description is for higher verte-brates.) With but few exceptions, it is voluntary muscle, i.e., under voluntary control. *Examples:* tongue muscle, biceps, triceps, and several hundred other muscles.

1. LONGITUDINAL SECTION
a. Parallel, cylindrical, eosinophilic fibers of about the same size.
b. Fibers of greater length and diameter than in smooth muscle.
c. *Cross-striations* (continuous, alternate dark and light bands).
d. *Numerous oval nuclei in close relation to sarcolemma.* Nuclei eccentric in position.
e. Interfibrous connective tissue nuclei present.

2. CROSS SECTION
a. Nearly all fibers the same size, eosinophilic.
b. Myofibrils visible as dots in groups (Cohnheim's fields) in the fibers.
c. *Nuclei infrequently seen in cross section, but when present usually appear to be placed in the "corners" of the fibers.* To be more exact, the nuclei are usually located directly under the cell membrane (sarcolemma). *The peripherally placed nuclei constitute the most diagnostic feature of transverse sections.*
d. Fibers appear rounded or polygonal in outline.
e. Fibers may be grouped in fasciculi with connective tissue between the fasciculi.

C. Cardiac Muscle

Since the fibers of cardiac muscle lie in various planes, *areas will be found in a single section in which they are cut both longitudinally and transversely.* They are compact in general appearance.

1. LONGITUDINAL SECTION
a. *Fibers branch and anastomose.*
b. Protoplasm granular and may show pigmentation.
c. *Large oval nuclei, usually near central axis of fibers.*
d. Region surrounding nucleus contains no myofibrils.
e. *Irregular cross-striations closer together and not so clearly visible as in skeletal muscle.*
f. Intercalated disks are cross bands peculiar to heart muscle. These disks are usually very indistinct in ordinary preparations, but may be brought out clearly with special staining techniques.

---

[1] Skeletal muscle is also called *striated,* but inasmuch as cardiac muscle too is striated, the use of the term *striated* for skeletal may result in some confusion.

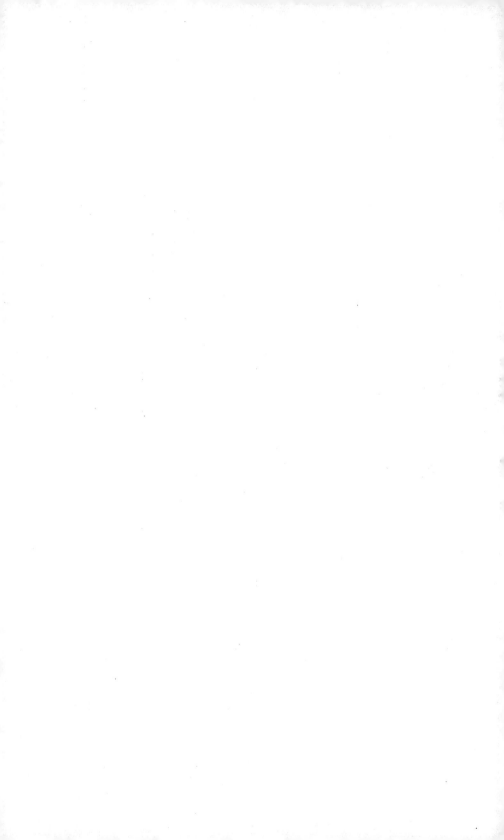

As shown by electron microscopy, they represent junctions between cells, the plasma membrane being modified to become much denser than elsewhere. The intercalated disks are structurally similar to desmosomes.

 g. Sarcolemma present, but a thinner sheath than surrounds skeletal muscle fibers.

2. CROSS SECTION

 a. *Nuclei relatively rare, more or less centrally placed in fibers.*

 b. No definite fasciculi.

 c. *Nuclei larger than in voluntary muscle.*

 d. Cut ends of myofibrils often show radial arrangement so as to suggest short parallel bands or spokes of a wheel.

 e. Purkinje fibers. Under the endocardium of the heart, particularly that of the interventricular septum, appears a net of atypical muscle fibers, Purkinje fibers; this network is made up of separate cellular units. The sarcoplasm of the Purkinje cells appears to be divided into separate sections. The Purkinje fibers have intercalated disks, and large amounts of sarcoplasm are accumulated about the nuclei. In many places a gradual transition of the Purkinje fibers to cardiac fibers may be noticed.

TABLE 4. SPECIAL FEATURES OF THE THREE TYPES OF MUSCLES, AS AN AID TO DIAGNOSIS

Type	Myofibrils	Nucleus	Sarcolemma	Shape and Size
Smooth:				
Cross section	Invisible	Central	Not distinct	Circular; 7 microns
Longitudinal section	Faint; no striations; vague markings	Central	Not distinct	Spindle-shaped
Skeletal:				
Cross section	Visible; grouped dots	Peripheral	Sheath is definite	Rounded, polygonal; 17–87 microns
Longitudinal section	Well-marked striations	Peripheral	Sheath is definite	Spindle-shaped
Cardiac:				
Cross section	Visible as dots; radial arrangement	Central	Sheath is thin	Round; 9–20 microns
Longitudinal section	Lightly striated; cross-striations	Central	Sheath is thin	Branching

Chapter 9 NERVOUS TISSUE

Nervous tissue is specialized for the reception of stimuli and the transmission of impulses to all parts of the body. This is the most highly specialized tissue in animals. The nervous system consists of the following tissues: nerve cells (neurons), supporting tissue (neuroglia), and the connective tissue proper, including the meninges and the coverings of the nerves.

A. Nerve Cells (Neurons)

1. **CYTOPLASM.** Part surrounding nucleus, sometimes called the *perikaryon*. In the axon it is termed *axoplasm*. A variety of techniques are necessary to demonstrate the various constituents; therefore several different preparations must be studied to observe the whole cytologic picture.

   a. NEUROFIBRILS. Threads which run in every direction and extend into the nerve processes.

   b. CHROMOPHIL SUBSTANCE (NISSL BODIES). Chromophil substance consists of discrete clumps in living cells. These clumps belong to the chromidial group in the system of endoplasmic reticulum. This group stains deeply with aniline dyes, much like the chromatin of the nucleus. Nissl bodies occur in dendrites, but are not present in the axon or at its point of implantation on the cell body (axon hillock). By electron microscopy they consist of ribonucleoprotein (RNP, ribosomes), which is both free and associated with the endoplasmic reticulum.

2. **NUCLEUS.** It is roughly spherical and relatively large, especially in the motor neurons of the ventral horns of the gray matter of the cord.

3. **NERVE PROCESSES.** A typical nerve cell has branched processes arising from the cell body. Three distinct types of nerve cells are recognized according to the number of processes which they possess.

   a. UNIPOLAR (MONOPOLAR) CELL. A single process, the *axon*, extends out from the cell body. It does not have dendritic

processes. In the vertebrate such neurons appear in early embryonic stages and in cerebrospinal ganglia.

b. BIPOLAR CELL. *Examples:* bipolar cells of the retina and in the cells which compose the spiral ganglion and vestibular ganglion of the acoustic nerve. Bipolar neurons give off two processes, one at either end of the cell body.

c. MULTIPOLAR CELL. *Example:* motor cells from the ventral horn of the spinal cord. Several processes consisting of one axon and a number of dendrites.

B. Myelinated (Medullated) Nerve Fibers

1. LONGITUDINAL SECTION OF FIBER

a. Parallel fibers, usually stain lightly.

b. Irregular diameter of fibers gives a section the general appearance of being wavy.

c. Neurilemma (neurolemma) cells with finely granular oval nuclei. These cells form a tubelike membrane.

d. *Central axis cylinder visible, composed of small delicate threads (neurofibrils).*

e. Nodes of Ranvier.

f. Schmidt-Lantermann clefts.

2. CROSS SECTION OF FIBER AND NERVE TRUNK

a. *Irregular small circles (the neurilemma) of different sizes, each with a dark, deeply stained dot (the axis cylinder).*

b. The space between the axis cylinder and the neurilemma (sheath of Schwann) corresponds to that occupied by the myelin in the living tissue.

c. In preparations stained only with osmic acid, the myelin sheath appears as a black ring enclosing the unstained axis cylinder, and both are enclosed by the neurilemma. By electron microscopy the myelin sheath represents concentric layers of plasma membrane formed as a result of the Schwann cell wrapping itself around the axis cylinder again and again.

d. There are three connective tissue sheaths which may be observed in a transverse section of a large nerve trunk.

(1) Epineurium. Outermost connective tissue sheath surrounding several fasciculi.

(2) Perineurium. Sheath around each individual fasciculus.

(3) Endoneurium. Prolongations of the perineurium extend as septa into the large nerve bundles, and may penetrate between individual nerve fibers.

C. **Unmyelinated (Nonmedullated) Nerve Fibers.** *Example:* nerves found between the circular and longitudinal layers of smooth muscle in any part of the digestive tube.

1. Very small and inconspicuous compared with myelinated fibers.
2. Viewed in cross section, the unmyelinated fibers appear as small discrete dots, which remain distinct with changing focus. In longitudinal sections, they look like fine parallel lines. Obliquely cut, they are difficult to recognize.
3. Axis cylinders composed of neurofibrils.
4. Axis cylinder usually covered by a delicate neurilemma.
5. *Their diameter is small, sometimes less than one micron.*
6. Compared with medullated fibers, they are very inconspicuous. They lie within the cytoplasm of the Schwann cell, but the Schwann cell does not surround them with plasma membrane as occurs in myelinated fibers.

D. **Cerebrospinal Ganglia**

1. *Cells appear round and granular and are larger than those of the autonomic ganglia.*
2. Nuclei are vesicular and may contain prominent nucleoli.
3. *Large bundles of nerve fibers may isolate cells into groups.*
4. *Large bundles of myelinated nerve fibers traverse the ganglion.*

E. **Autonomic Ganglia**

1. *Cell bodies are usually smaller and have somewhat more irregular contours than those of the cerebrospinal ganglia.*
2. Nuclei are located eccentrically in the cell body, whereas in cerebrospinal ganglia, they are located centrally.
3. *No definite grouping of cells in the autonomic ganglia.*
4. Capsule is less distinct and contains less satellite cells than does the capsule of a cerebrospinal ganglion cell.
5. Autonomic ganglia do not show the regular arrangement of large bundles of myelinated fibers traversing the ganglion.
6. *Chiefly nonmedullated fibers lining the ganglion.*

F. **Motor Nerve Endings.** Special staining techniques are required to demonstrate these structures.

1. **MOTOR NERVE ENDINGS OF STRIATED MUSCLES**
   a. *Nerves end in motor end plates.*
   b. Each nerve just before ending becomes much branched so as to innervate from 10 to 20 muscle fibers.

2. MOTOR NERVE ENDINGS OF SMOOTH AND CARDIAC MUSCLES

a. Nerve terminations more simple than in striated muscle.
b. Repeated branching forms a *primary plexus,* which surrounds the muscle bundles.
c. Axis cylinder fibers from primary plexus may penetrate the smooth muscle or cardiac muscle to form a delicate *secondary plexus,* from which short branches pass to end in minute dilations or granules on the muscle cells.

G. **Sensory Nerve Endings (Afferent Receptors).** These endings are homologues of dendrites as distinguished from the motor end plates which are equivalent to axon endings. The sensory endings vary in structures as follows:

1. NONENCAPSULATED ENDINGS

a. Free endings are the simplest type and occur in epithelium, connective tissue, muscle, and serous membranes. The branches end in varicose or minute granules.
b. Merkel's disks (corpuscles of Merkel). *Examples:* deep layers of epithelium of the skin and external root sheath of hair. Skin of duck's bill is good material for study.
  (1) Consists of expanded disks of terminal twigs of the branches of nerve fibers which penetrate stratified squamous epithelium.
  (2) Tactile in function.

2. ENCAPSULATED ENDINGS

a. Pacinian corpuscles (corpuscles of vater-pacini, lamellar corpuscles). *Examples:* penis, clitoris, nipple, mammary gland, conjunctiva, cornea, heart, mesentery, pancreas, deeper subcutaneous connective tissue, and in loose connective tissue generally.
  (1) Elliptical in shape. Often as large as a pin head and easily seen by the unaided eye.
  (2) *Inner core (bulb) surrounded by lamellae of connective tissue. In cross section, the lamellae look like the concentric rings in a freshly cut tree trunk.*
  (3) The inner core contains the termination of the nerve fiber.
b. Touch corpuscles of meissner (tactile corpuscles) *Example:* in connective tissue papillae of the skin.
  (1) Corpuscle has peculiar spirally striated appearance.
  (2) Within corpuscle, nerve fibers break into a plexus of varicose fibers, many of which end in knobbed extremities.
  (3) Corpuscles surrounded by connective tissue capsule.

c. MUSCLE SPINDLES (NEUROMUSCULAR BUNDLES)
   (1) Groups of poorly differentiated muscle fibers enclosed within a connective tissue sheath.
   (2) The sheath is perforated by one or more sensory nerve fibers which end around the muscle fibers.
   (3) The muscle fibers of the spindle are thinner than ordinary fibers. They also contain more nuclei, especially in the regions surrounded by nerve fibers.
   (4) Identification of neuromuscular spindles is of special importance to pathologists, since the spindles persist after all contractile elements have undergone atrophy or have been replaced by adipose tissue. Hence, the muscle spindles provide a valuable means of recognizing a region of muscle tissue under extreme pathologic conditions.
d. MUSCLE-TENDON SPINDLES (ORGANS OF GOLGI)
   (1) Located at junction of muscle with tendon.
   (2) The spindle consists of tendon bundles usually covered by a thin capsule.
   (3) One or several afferent nerve fibers enter the spindle, where they break into complicated arborizations.

H. **Neuroglia ("Glia").** This constitutes the supporting tissue of the central nervous system, of the retina, and of the capsular cells of the peripheral ganglia. The neuroglia cells, though supportive in function, are usually considered with the conductive elements of the nervous system. Cytoplasm and processes can be seen only by special histologic techniques.

1. ASTROCYTES FROM ECTODERM
   a. Cell bodies with innumerable long slender processes.
      (1) Protoplasmic Astrocytes. These are *short-rayed astrocytes,* which have a *mossy appearance.* Some of the processes end in perivascular feet.
      (2) Fibrous Astrocytes. These are *long-rayed astrocytes,* which do not branch as extensively as the protoplasmic astrocytes and are *spiderlike.* Also perivascular feet which clasp blood vessels.

2. OLIGODENDROCYTES (OLIGODENDROGLIA) FROM ECTODERM
   a. Cells and nuclei small. Processes are *fine and few as compared with astrocytes.*

3. MICROGLIA FROM MESODERM
   a. Very small, elongated cell bodies with deeply staining nuclei, *beset with spines.*

4. EPENDYMA

   a. Closely packed columnar epithelial cells lying in the thick walled portions of the ventricles of the brain.
   b. The axes of the cells are perpendicular to the central canal and ventricles.
   c. The cells may have cilia which protrude into the neural cavity in certain forms and in certain places.

I. Spinal Cord

1. *Composed of a central column of gray matter which is roughly H-shaped in cross section.* Motor nerve cells are grouped in the larger lobes of the "H," which are termed the ventral or anterior horns. In center of cord is ependyma-lined central canal.
2. *White matter surrounding the gray matter is composed of transversely cut nerve fibers of ascending and descending tracts.*
3. Surface may show pia, a thin connective tissue layer with blood vessels.

J. Cerebellum

1. The cortex consists of three layers:
   a. An outer molecular layer of few cells and many nonmedullated fibers.
   b. An intermediate (middle) single ganglionic layer composed of *Purkinje cells (treelike).*
   c. An inner granular layer or nuclear layer that consists of the bodies of small nerve cells.

K. Cerebrum

1. Light-staining background with many small fibers and a few small round nuclei.
2. *Various-sized pyramidal cells; sometimes perineuronal spaces are made conspicuous by shrinkage of the cells.*
3. The cerebral cortex, generally speaking, exhibits six layers. The amount of development of these six layers differs in different areas. The six layers are from without inward:
   a. MOLECULAR (ZONAL LAYER, PLEXIFORM LAYER). This layer contains horizontal cells; some cells with short axons; terminal branches of apical dendrite of pyramidal cells.
   b. OUTER GRANULAR LAYER. The dendrites of this layer in the main enter the first layer; axons pass downward into white matter.
   c. PYRAMIDAL CELL LAYER. This layer is composed of typical

pyramids sending dendrite branches into first layer and axons into white matter. It also contains many granule cells with short axons and Martinotti's cells.

d. INNER GRANULAR LAYER. Predominantly stellar cells in this layer; the larger of these sending their axons into white matter. Many short axon granules present.

e. GANGLIONIC OR INTERNAL PYRAMIDAL LAYER. Large- and medium-sized pyramids. They send axons into white matter. Short axons and Martinotti's cells.

f. MULTIFORM LAYER. Polymorphic or fusiform cells. Spindle-shaped cells which send axons into white matter. Outer zone has larger cells more densely packed; inner zone smaller cells, loosely arranged. Also short axons and Martinotti's cells.

4. White matter lies below the cerebral cortex. This consists of inter-lacing bundles of myelinated fibers.

Chapter 10   THE CIRCULATORY SYSTEM

The circulatory system consists of the heart, blood vessels, and lymphatics. It sends nutrients, oxygen, and hormones to all parts of the body and carries wastes from the tissues to the kidneys.

The division of blood vessels into various types is artificial for one type of vessel merges into another without marked boundaries. Sometimes arteries of rather small caliber have walls which suggest large arteries, and vice versa. *In general, veins can be distinguished from arteries of the same size by a thinner wall; hence, in sections, veins which are empty, appear collapsed, and their lumens are irregular and slitlike.*

A. Capillaries. Vary in diameter from 4.5 to 12.0 microns. Capillaries consist of endothelium, basement membrane, and pericytes (Rouget cells). Some capillaries may contain fenestrations in the endothelium as capillaries of the kidney and endocrine organs.

  1. They connect arterioles and venules.

  2. Capillaries are endothelial tubes usually separated from other tissues by a thin connective tissue layer. Some authors consider the delicate connective sheath around these endothelial tubes to be an elementary adventitia.

  3. Walls only one cell layer in thickness.

B. Small Arteries (Arterioles). Arteries with a caliber of 0.3 mm or less.

  1. *Tunica intima* consists of endothelium and the internal elastic membrane. *The latter is markedly scalloped in sections.*

  2. *Tunica media consists of smooth muscle fibers.*

  3. *Tunica adventitia (externa)* approximately equals the media in thickness; it is a layer of loose connective tissue with longitudinally oriented, thin, collagenous, and elastic fibers. Small arteries lack a definite external membrane.

C. Medium-sized Arteries (Muscular Type). *Example:* radial artery.

  1. Tunica intima similar to above except that it is thicker. This is due to a layer which consists of a few fibroblasts, thin collagenous

bundles, and thin interlacing elastic fibers between the endothelium and the internal elastic membrane.

2. *Tunica media differs from that of arteriole, not only by possessing a thicker muscle layer, but also by possessing thin elastic fibers which appear between the cells as the caliber of the vessel increases.*

3. Tunica adventitia, comparatively *very thick,* and sometimes thicker than the tunica media. An external elastic membrane, immediately adjacent to the smooth muscles, stands out well defined.

D. Large-sized Arteries (Elastic Type). *Example:* aorta.

1. Tunica intima is relatively thick. Thin subendothelial layer is bound externally by a fenestrated elastic membrane. Poorly delimited from the tunica media because of the large amount of elastic tissue in the media, forming membranes similar to the internal elastic membrane of the intima.

2. *Tunica media consists mainly of elastic tissue.*

3. Tunica adventitia is relatively thin. Like the tunica intima, it cannot be sharply distinguished from the media because of the absence of a well-defined, external, elastic membrane which is different from the most external of the elastic membranes of the media. There is a gradual transition from the tunica adventitia into the surrounding, loose, irregularly arranged, connective tissue which contains many fat cells. In the adventitia and outer portion of the media are small blood vessels (*vasa vasorum*) and nerves (*nervi vasorum*).

E. Arteriovenous Anastomoses

1. In different parts of the body, many arterioles connect directly with venules instead of through capillaries, especially in limbs and exposed parts of the body; this is probably a function in temperature control.

2. As an arteriole passes to a venule, the subendothelial elastic tissue disappears and the endothelium lies directly upon the musculature.

3. The whole of the vessel has a thickened adventitia of loose collagenous connective tissue.

4. Arteriovenous anastomoses look more like an arteriole with a thickened wall than a venule.

F. Coccygeal Body (Glomus Coccygeum)

This organ, sometimes incorrectly included in the paraganglia, does not contain chromaffin cells.

1. Located in front of the apex of the coccyx, and 2.5 mm in diameter.

2. It consists of numerous arteriovenous anastomoses with a relatively thick muscle wall embedded in dense fibrous connective tissue.
3. The modified *smooth muscle cells of the vessel walls resemble epithelioid cells, giving an endocrine appearance.*

G. Small Veins

1. Diameter of about 20 microns.
   a. These consist of a layer of *endothelium surrounded by a very thin layer of connective tissue* composed of longitudinally directed collagenous fibers and fibroblasts.
2. Diameter of about 45–200 microns.
   a. Smooth muscle cells appear between endothelium and connective tissue when the diameter increases to about 45 microns. At this diameter the muscle cells are some distance from each other; they later become arranged closer and closer together until a continuous layer is present in veins with a diameter of about 200 microns.
3. Diameter of over 200 microns.
   a. Tunica intima consists only of endothelium.
   b. Tunica media consists of one or *several layers of smooth muscle cells.*
   c. Tunica adventitia consists of scattered fibroblasts and thin elastic and collagenous fibers.

H. Medium-sized Veins. Diameter of from 2 to 9 mm.

1. Tunica intima has a peculiar endothelium in that its cells, in contrast to the elongated cells of the arteries, are of polygonal form; sometimes an inconspicuous connective tissue layer is present which contains more or less elastic fibers. Tunica intima is poorly developed in comparison to that of an artery. A distinct boundary between intima and media may not exist.
2. *Tunica media is much thinner than in the arteries.* It consists *mainly of circularly arranged, smooth muscle fibers,* between which are abundant, longitudinal, collagenous fibers.
3. Tunica adventitia is usually much thicker than the media. It consists of *irregularly arranged connective tissue with rather thick, longitudinal, collagenous bundles* and elastic network. Adjacent to the media there may be some smooth muscle fibers.

I. Large-sized Veins

1. Tunica intima has same structure as in the medium-sized veins.
2. *Tunica media has varying thicknesses; in general, it is poorly de-*

veloped and is sometimes absent. The structure is the same as that in veins of medium caliber.

3. *Tunica adventitia composes the greater part of the venous wall and is usually several times the thickness of the media.* It consists of irregularly arranged connective tissues containing thick elastic fibers, and, mainly, longitudinal collagenous fibers. Adjacent to the media, or to the intima if the former is absent, the adventitia contains very well-developed longitudinal layers of smooth muscles and elastic networks.

4. The blood vessels of the blood vessels (*vasa vasorum*) are more abundant in veins than in arteries.

5. Valves are present in many veins, especially in the extremities.
   a. They consist of projections of the intima in the form of semi-lunar flaps with the concavity directed toward the heart.
   b. The flaps (leaflets) are composed of connective tissue covered with endothelium.

J. Sinusoids

In some organs such as the adrenal and bone marrow, instead of capillaries, sinusoids are interposed between the arterial and venous sides of the circulation.

1. Structurally, the sinusoids differ from capillaries in the following ways:
   a. *They usually have a larger lumen (5–30 microns in diameter) with irregular tortuous walls.*
   b. Thin endothelial lining may be incomplete.
   c. Sinusoids are accompanied by a dense membranous network of reticular fibrils.
   d. The basement membrane of sinusoids is incomplete or absent.
   e. Some of the lining cells of sinusoids may be phagocytic.

2. In the adult mammalian body, sinusoids occur in the erectile tissue of male and female genitalia, in the parathyroids, spleen, liver, and other viscera.

K. Lymphatic Vessels

1. *Lymphatic vessels are to be distinguished from veins of the same size, not only by their decidedly thinner walls and more collapsed appearance, but also by absence of red corpuscles in lumen of the vessel unless extravasation has occurred. On the other hand, lymphocytes are frequently present, together with a granular or fibrous coagulum. The tissue is loosely arranged as compared with that of a vein.*

Cross sections of cat intestine, in the phase of fat absorption, stained with Sudan III, give a striking demonstration of lymphatic vessels.

2. Small lymphatic vessels are difficult to distinguish from inter-fibrillar tissue spaces because of their collapsed condition. *Lymphatic capillaries may appear as endothelium-lined irregular spaces in the connective tissue.*

3. As the lymphatic vessels become larger they are covered by thin, mainly collagenous bundles, elastic fibers, and a few smooth muscle cells. Those lymphatic vessels with a diameter greater than 0.2 mm have thick walls composed of three layers: *intima, media,* and *adventitia.* The boundaries between these layers are often indistinct.

4. The thoracic duct possesses a muscular media thicker than a vein of the same size.

5. Valves occur in pairs placed on the opposite sides within the lymph vessel. They prevent the lymph from reversing its direction.

L. Heart

The heart is composed of three layers: the *endocardium,* the *myocardium,* and the *epicardium.* The first is continuous with the intima of the blood vessels; the myocardium (muscular layer) corresponds to the media, and the epicardium to the adventitia except that its outer surface is covered with mesothelium.

1. ATRIA

a. Endocardium is thicker in the atria, especially in the left atrium, than in the ventricles.

b. *Myocardium much thinner than in the ventricles.*

2. RIGHT VENTRICLE

a. *Compact part about one-third of entire thickness. Looser part (columna carneae) about two-thirds.*

3. LEFT VENTRICLE

a. *Compact part two-thirds, loose part one-third of entire thickness.*

b. Myocardium thickest in the left ventricle.

4. PAPILLARY MUSCLE

a. Small area of heart muscle surrounded by endothelial cells (endocardium).

5. CHORDA TENDINEA

a. *Composed of collagenous and elastic fibers surrounded by endocardium (endothelial cells).*

b. Any of the heart sections may show epicardium or endocardium.

6. VALVES

a. The valves of the heart are folds of endocardium.

b. Atrioventricular valves consist of fibrous and elastic tissue. Although smooth muscle fibers are found on the atrial side of the valves, they are not likely to be observed except in specially prepared slides.

c. Aortic and pulmonary valves are similar to those above, but contain no muscle fibers.

7. IMPULSE CONDUCTING SYSTEM

a. Atrioventricular bundle of His consists of strands of fibers that are larger than cardiac muscle fibers. First described by Purkinje, hence often called Purkinje fibers. These cardiac muscle fibers are not rich in myofibrils, and in most preparations contain large empty spaces due to extracted or unstained glycogen. These fibers are subendocardial.

b. Sinoatrial and atrioventricular nodes consist of a network of fibers whose meshes are filled with connective tissue.

TABLE 5. SUMMARY OF THE HISTOLOGY OF THE CIRCULATORY SYSTEM

Blood Vessels	Endothelium	Connective Tissue	Muscle	Tunica Intima (Interna)	Tunica Media	Tunica Adventitia (Externa)
Capillaries About 8 microns	Present	Thin layer usually separates them from other tissue	None	None	None	Pericytes
Small Arteries (Arterioles) 0.3 mm or smaller	Present	Elastic and collagenous fibers	Smooth	Endothelium and internal elastic membrane	Smooth muscle fibers	Loose connective tissue with longitudinally oriented elastic and collagenous fibers
Medium-sized Arteries (Muscular type)	Present	Elastic and collagenous fibers	Smooth	Between endothelium and internal elastic membrane a few fibroblasts; elastic and collagenous fibers in larger vessels of this caliber	Thick muscle layer; as caliber increases thin elastic fibers appear between cells	Sometimes thicker than tunica media; external elastic membrane adjacent to media well defined; loose connective tissue with elastic and collagenous fibers
Large-sized Arteries (Elastic type)	Present	Elastic and collagenous fibers	Smooth muscle fibers present but not abundant	Rather thick; fibroblasts, collagenous and elastic fibers present; a few smooth muscle cells may be present	Mainly of elastic tissue	Relatively thin; consists of elastic and collagenous tissue

Arteries

98

Blood Vessels	Endothelium	Connective Tissue	Muscle	Tunica Intima (Interna)	Tunica Media	Tunica Adventitia (Externa)
Small Veins (Venules) About 20 microns	Present	Longitudinally directed collagenous fibers and fibroblasts surround endothelium	None	None	None	None
About 45 microns	Present	Elastic and collagenous fibers	Smooth muscle cells between endothelium and connective tissue	None	None	None
Over 200 microns	Present	Elastic and collagenous fibers	Smooth	Endothelium	Several layers of smooth muscle cells	Scattered fibroblasts and thin elastic and collagenous fibers
Medium-sized Veins 2-9 mm	Present	Elastic and collagenous fibers	Circular smooth muscle	Endothelium; sometimes inconspicuous connective tissue layer present	Mainly of circular smooth muscles between which are abundant longitudinal, collagenous fibers	Loose connective tissue with collagenous bundles and elastic networks
Large-sized Veins	Present	Elastic and collagenous fibers	Smooth	Endothelium; sometimes inconspicuous connective tissue layer present	Sometimes absent; when present mainly of circular smooth muscles between which are abundant, longitudinal, collagenous fibers	Loose connective tissue containing elastic and mainly longitudinal collagenous fibers; adjacent to media, or, if absent, to intima, longitudinal layers of smooth muscles, and elastic networks

Veins

99

TABLE 5. SUMMARY OF THE HISTOLOGY OF THE CIRCULATORY SYSTEM (Continued)

Blood Vessels	Endothelium	Connective Tissue	Muscle	Tunica Intima (Interna)	Tunica Media	Tunica Adventitia (Externa)
Sinusoids 5–30 microns	May be incomplete	Little or none	None	None	None	None
Lymphatic Capillaries	Present	None	None	None	None	None
Lymphatic Vessels Less than 0.2 mm	Present	Mainly longitudinal, collagenous, and elastic fibers	A few smooth muscle cells	None	None	None
Lymphatic Vessels More than 0.2 mm	Present	Elastic and collagenous fibers	Smooth	Endothelium and thin layer of longitudinal elastic fibers	Several layers of mainly circular smooth muscles interspersed with elastic fibers	Interlacing collagenous and elastic fibers, and smooth muscle fibers

Chapter 11   LYMPHATIC (LYMPHOID) ORGANS

Reticular tissue, lymphocytes, and related cells constitute the lymphatic tissue proper of the so-called lymphatic organs.

A. Lymph Nodes

1. Generally round or oval.
2. Capsule of dense collagenous and elastic connective tissue.
3. Cortex.
   a. Subcapsular (cortical, peripheral) sinus appears as a pale-staining area which lies immediately beneath the capsule.
   b. *Cortex contains nodules with germinal centers. Small arteries in nodules not sheathed as in spleen.*
4. Medulla.
   a. Medullary cords consist of dense lymphatic tissue which stains darkly.
   b. Cords are surrounded by sinuses which appear as light-colored areas.
   c. Afferent lymphatic vessels pierce the capsule at its periphery. At one point the capsule is indented and thickened. This is the hilus and it is from here that the efferent lymphatic vessels emerge.
5. *Pulmonary and bronchial lymphatic tissues commonly contain considerable carbon particles.*

B. Hemal (Hemolymph) Nodes

1. Typical hemal node resembles a lymph node in its general structure.
2. Covered by a connective tissue capsule from which a very few trabeculae enter the node.
3. When nodules with germinal centers are present they are usually found in the cortex.
4. Entirely devoid of lymphatic vessels.
5. *Sinuses filled with erythrocytes.*

6. There is some question as to whether hemal nodes are constant structures in man.

C. Spleen

1. The spleen is much like a large lymph node, but the fibromuscular capsule is thicker and the trabeculae are larger. The external surface of the capsule is covered by mesothelium.
2. *Fibromuscular trabeculae, which extend from the periphery into the substance of the organ, tend to be at right angles to the capsule.* Their presence is the most distinctive characteristic as the fibromuscular trabeculae persist after all other features disappear under pathologic conditions.
3. Splenic pulp is divided into two varieties as follows:
   a. Red pulp contains primitive reticular cells, lymphocytes, free macrophages, and all types of cells found in the circulating blood and venous sinuses. *Erythrocytes give the characteristic red color to this part of the organ.*
   b. White pulp surrounds arteries and includes splenic nodules. This contains primitive reticular cells, fixed macrophages, and large numbers of lymphocytes. *The areas of white pulp stain a deep purple in preparations dyed with hematoxylin and eosin.*
4. *Splenic nodules (Malpighian bodies, splenic corpuscles) with so-called central arteries are very diagnostic in the higher vertebrates.*
5. *No division into cortex and medulla.*

D. Thymus

1. YOUNG

a. Subdivided into lobes by connective tissue. These lobes subsequently divided into lobules.
b. *Each lobule has a definitely darker cortex and a lighter medulla. Each lobule resembles a lymph node, but germinal centers are not present and no lymph sinuses are found.*
c. *Only medulla contains thymic (Hassall's) corpuscles* which are eosinophilic and show an arrangement of concentric layers. Occasionally they are lacking.
d. *Medulla does not have cords of cells* and trabeculae as do the lymph nodes.
e. *No nodules in cortex,* but cortex consists of densely packed small lymphocytes which are termed *thymocytes* by some authors.

2. ATROPHIC

a. *Adipose tissue with strands of lymphatic tissue.*

(1) These strands contain thymic corpuscles. The corpuscles are generally larger in old thymus. The clearly lobulated structure is lost, as is the cortex and medulla arrangement.

E. Tonsil. In tonsil tissue the epithelium is usually so infiltrated with lymphocytes that it stains darker and is less distinct than usual. A tonsil possesses no sinuses either for blood or for lymph.

1. LINGUAL TONSILS
    a. *No definite fibrous tissue capsule.*
    b. Covered on free surface by a stratified squamous epithelium.
    c. *Relatively shallow, slightly branching crypts, lined with stratified squamous epithelium.*
    d. Crypts surrounded by lymphatic nodules with germinal centers. Clear central germinating area surrounded by a darker area of smaller, more compact cells. Few crypts as compared with palatine tonsil.
    e. Tongue muscles and mucous glands which lie beneath the lingual tonsil may be associated with the tonsil in sections.

2. PALATINE TONSILS
    a. Covered on free surface by a stratified squamous epithelium. Epithelium may be infiltrated with lymphocytes.
    b. *Contain many deep-branched crypts (10–20), and, when sectioned, oval or slitlike isolated spaces lined with stratified squamous epithelium often appear.*
    c. Crypts surrounded by many lymph nodules.
    d. Exudate commonly found in crypts.
    e. Crypts are partly separated from one another by partitions of loose connective tissue.
    f. *A definite fibrous connective tissue capsule invests the portion of the gland which is not bordered by epithelium.*
    g. Striated muscle which is frequently found external to the connective tissue of the capsule of a vertical section is evidence of the close relation of the tonsil to the underlying muscular structures.
    h. Cartilage plates may be present in old hypertrophied tonsils.

3. PHARYNGEAL TONSILS
    a. Like palatine (faucial) tonsils except:
        (1) *Less definite capsule.*
        (2) Free surface covered for most part by pseudostratified ciliated epithelium; however, there may be patches of stratified squamous epithelium. Epithelium infiltrated with many lymphocytes.

(3) Crypts generally absent but numerous folds lined with pseudostratified ciliated epithelium.

(4) If crypts present, may be lined with pseudostratified epithelium.

4. TUBAL TONSILS

a. Small accumulations of lymphatic tissue located about the openings of the Eustachian tubes into the pharynx.

TABLE 6. SUMMARY OF THE HISTOLOGY OF THE LYMPHATIC ORGANS

Organ	Capsule	Hilus	Cortex	Medulla	Epithelium	Lymphatic Nodules	Lymphatic Vessels	Lymphatic Sinuses
Lymph Nodes	Connective tissue and smooth muscle fibers	Present	Nodules and diffuse lymphatic tissue	Medullary cords of dense lymphatic tissue	None	Present in cortex	Afferent and efferent	Peripheral and medullary
Hemal Nodes	Connective tissue	Present	Irregular masses; nodules may be present	Anastomosing cords of tissue	None	Present	None	None; sinuses contain blood
Spleen	Elastic and collagenous fibers; a few muscle cells present	Present	None	None	Mesothelium	Around central artery	Only in capsule and trabeculae	None
Thymus	Connective tissue	None	Densely packed cells	Hassall's corpuscles	Present	None	Penetrate lymphatic tissue	None
Lingual Tonsil	No definite fibrous tissue capsule	None	None	None	Stratified squamous	With germinal centers; clustered around crypts	None	None
Palatine Tonsil	Definite fibrous tissue capsule	None	None	None	Stratified squamous	Surround crypts; usually in a single layer under the epithelium	None	None
Pharyngeal Tonsil	Less definite than in palatine tonsil	None	None	None	Pseudostratified ciliated and stratified squamous	Surround crypts	None	None
Tubal Tonsils	See page 108							

Tonsils

110

Chapter 12

SKIN AND ITS APPENDAGES

A. Skin (Integument)

It consists of an epidermis of ectodermal origin and a dermis (corium) of mesodermal origin. It rests on a layer of connective tissue.

1. **EPIDERMIS.** This is a stratified squamous epithelium. Its thickness varies with the region of the body; it is thickest on the palms of the hands and the soles of the feet. Two layers, lucidum and granulosum, are usually absent in thin skin.
   a. In thick skin the following layers, from within outward, can be distinguished.
   (1) Stratum Germinativum (Malpighian Layer). *It is deeply basophilic and the nuclei are prominent.* This layer can be divided into two sublayers as follows.
   (a) Basal layer (Stratum cylindricum). Consists of a single row of columnar cells with indistinct outlines. It gives rise to the layers above. Mitotic figures are frequently observed.
   (b) Spiny layer (Stratum spinosum). The cells are polygonal. They are somewhat flattened in the superficial layers. They seem connected with each other by protoplasmic intercellular bridges which appear as spines on individual cells. For this reason the cells are called "prickle cells." The intercellular bridges are actually apposed modified aspects of the plasma membrane as is shown by electron microscopy. There is no actual continuity from cell to cell. The "prickle cells" are difficult to demonstrate in normal skin, but show up well in certain mucous membranes, skin warts, and cancers.
   (2) Stratum Granulosum (Granular Layer). *It consists of somewhat flattened cells, the cytoplasm of which contains a number of coarse, deeply staining granules of keratohyalin.* Intercellular bridges are present but difficult to observe.

In ordinary preparations of vertical sections, the cells appear to be separated by narrow spaces so that each is surrounded by a light line.

(3) Stratum Lucidum. A thin clear layer with indistinct nuclei and cell boundaries. *In sections the lucidum appears as a pale wavy stripe.*

(4) Stratum Corneum. *A thick, poorly staining layer of progressively flattened and cornified (keratinized, horny) cells which possess no nuclei.*

2. **DERMIS (DERMA, CORIUM).** The dermis roughly corresponds in thickness to the epidermis.

a. The dermis consists of two layers of collagenous and elastic fibers which are from without inward:

(1) Papillary Layer. It is not sharply demarked from the reticular layer. Structures supported by this layer of the dermis are (1) hairs and hair follicles, (2) sebaceous glands, (3) sweat glands, (4) blood vessels, and (5) nerves. It is called a papillary layer because the papillae are a prominent part of it.

(2) Reticular Layer. A layer composed of *coarser fibers* than the papillary layer; the fibers interlace with each other to form a network, hence the name reticular. It merges with the subcutaneous tissue.

3. **SUBCUTANEOUS TISSUE (HYPODERMIS, TELA SUBCUTANEA, SUBCUTIS)**

a. As the name implies, this layer is not a part of the skin proper. It serves to attach the skin to the deep fascia, muscles, and bones.

b. It consists of widely separated bundles of fibroelastic tissues and masses (lobules) of fat cells which occupy the spaces between them.

4. **PIGMENTATION.** The color of the human skin depends chiefly on the presence of pigments. It is said that the human skin contains four different pigments: (1) melanin, (2) oxyhemoglobin, (3) reduced hemoglobin, and (4) carotene. No additional pigments are found in the darker races, the differences in color being due to the amounts of various pigments.

B. Skin of the Scrotum

The skin of the scrotum has unique characteristics which merit special mention.

1. It possesses all the characteristics of thin skin; but, in addition,

there are coarse scattered bundles of smooth muscle in the reticular layer of the dermis. While these scattered bundles of smooth muscle are very characteristic of the scrotum, they are also found in the nipple, prepuce, glans penis, and in the perianal region. The contraction of these muscle fibers gives the skin of these regions its wrinkled appearance.

2. Especially rich in pigment are certain other patches of skin such as the axillae, areolae, nipples, labia majora, and the circumanal region.

C. Hair

Hairs are elastic horny threads developed from the epidermis. They grow within deep narrow pits (hair follicles) in the dermis which may extend into the subcutaneous tissue. Each hair consists of a shaft and a root which occupy the hair follicle.

The lower end of the root expands into a knoblike structure, the hair bulb.

1. **HAIR STRUCTURE.** Hair is made up entirely of epithelial cells which form three layers. They are, from within outward:

    a. MEDULLA. This forms the core of the hair. It consists of two or three layers of cuboidal cells whose crytoplasm stains lightly. The medulla does not extend the whole length of the hair; therefore, it is not observed in all sections.

    b. CORTEX. It makes up the main bulk of the hair. It is composed of several layers of spindle-shaped cells with shrunken nuclei. In colored hair, pigment is found between the cells of this layer.

    c. CUTICLE. An exceedingly thin layer composed of a single layer of scalelike overlapping cells, nucleated in the deeper parts of the sheath, nonnucleated near the surface.

2. **FOLLICLE STRUCTURE.** The follicle consists of the internal and external root sheaths derived from the epidermis, and an external connective tissue sheath derived from the dermis.

    a. INTERNAL ROOT SHEATH (INNER ROOT SHEATH). It consists of three distinct layers which are from within outward: (1) cuticle of the root sheath; (2) Huxley's layer (one to three layers of cells); and (3) Henle's layer (single row of somewhat flattened cells).

    b. EXTERNAL ROOT SHEATH (OUTER ROOT SHEATH). It is a continuation of the stratum germinativum. It consists of one to several layers of cells; the outermost row is composed of rather tall cells (stratum cylindricum).

    c. CONNECTIVE TISSUE SHEATH (THECA). It is a condensation of the dermis.

(1) Inner Layer. Really a hyaline membrane between the epithelial tissue and the connective tissue proper.

(2) Middle Layer. Consists óf circular bundles of connective tissue.

(3) Outer Layer. A poorly defined layer of loosely woven bundles of collagenous and elastic fibers which run longitudinally.

d. HAIR MATRIX. Consists of a mass of epithelial cells. The multiplication of these cells causes the hair to grow in length.

e. HAIR PAPILLA. A vascular extension of connective tissue which penetrates into the enlarged hair bulb.

f. ARRECTORES PILI (HAIR MUSCLE). Minute smooth muscle fibers, which arise from the papillary layer of the skin, and are inserted in the connective tissue sheath about the middle of the follicle.

D. Glands of Skin

Sebaceous, sweat, and mammary glands are all derived from the skin. Mammary glands are described in the section which deals with the female reproductive system.

1. **SEBACEOUS GLANDS.** Usually associated with a hair follicle, but in exceptional cases, such as in the corners of the mouth, on the mammary papillae, and elsewhere, they open directly on the surface of the skin.

    a. TYPE OF GLAND AND SHAPE. Simple or branched alveolar glands. They are spherical or ovoid in shape.

    b. STRUCTURE. The sebaceous glands appear as large, light-staining, solid islands of polyhedral cells with many vacuoles in their cytoplasm. Ducts usually empty obliquely into hair follicles. Each gland is surrounded by a fibrous sheath.

2. **SWEAT GLANDS.** They are found over the entire body surface, except in the eardrum, the nail bed, the margin of the lips, the inner surface of the prepuce, and the glans penis. They are the only glands found on palms of the hands and soles of the feet.

    a. TYPE OF GLANDS. Long, simple, coiled, tubular glands. *In sections they can be recognized as nests of small cut tubules.*

    b. WALLS OF SECRETORY PORTION, from without inward:

    (1) Basement Membrane.

    (2) Myoepithelial Cells. Flattened spindle-shaped cells. They are contractile and develop from ectoderm.

    (3) Gland Cells. They are cuboidal or low columnar, the height varying with activity.

c. Excretory Duct. These ducts have walls of two layers of cuboidal epithelium, which stains more deeply than the secretory cells. As the duct passes through the epidermis, its only walls are the cells of the epidermal layer.

E. Nails

The nails are modifications of the epidermis.

1. **NAIL BODY (NAILPLATE).** This is the exposed portion of the nail, and consists of closely welded horny scales, which are cornified epithelial cells.
2. **NAIL BED.** This is the skin under the body of the nail.
3. **NAIL ROOT.** The posterior part of the nail which lies under the skin.
4. **MATRIX.** This is the thickened germinativum which lies beneath the nail root. Growth of the nail results from a transformation of the superficial cells of the matrix into true nail cells.
5. **LUNULA.** This is the crescent-shaped white area of the nail near its root. It is seen best on the thumb. It is white because capillaries under it do not show through.
6. **NAIL WALL.** Consists of a fold of skin which surrounds the nail bed laterally and proximally.
7. **EPONYCHIUM.** This is the stratum corneum of the adjoining skin. It spreads over the upper surface of the nail root and forms what the layman calls *cuticle.*
8. **HYPONYCHIUM.** This is the thickened stratum corneum of the skin just beneath the free edge of the nail.

Chapter 13   DIGESTIVE SYSTEM

The digestive system consists of the alimentary canal proper, a tube extending from the mouth to the anus; and accessory structures such as the teeth, tongue, and glands. The wall of the alimentary canal, from the pharyngoesophageal junction to the rectoanal junction, has a common structural plan which is from within outward: (1) mucosa; (2) submucosa; (3) muscularis; and (4) either serosa, covering almost all the canal below the diaphragm, or adventitia, forming the external coat of the esophagus and part of the rectum.

A. Lips (Vertical Section)

The layers from without inward are:

1. **SKIN ON THE OUTSIDE.** It consists of stratified squamous epithelium which is keratinized at the surface, and rests on a layer of connective tissue.
2. **CONNECTIVE TISSUE.** In this are sweat glands, sebaceous glands, and the bases of hair follicles.
3. **STRIATED MUSCLE.** Muscles of the lip consist of the orbicularis and the mimetic.
4. **ORAL SURFACE**
   a. MUCOUS MEMBRANE. Like the lining of the soft parts of the oral cavity.
5. **TRANSITION FROM SKIN TO MUCOUS MEMBRANE**
   a. The transition from skin to oral mucosa is marked by the following characteristics.
   (1) Epithelium becomes gradually thicker.
   (2) Gradual disappearance of keratinized cells.
   (3) The height of the connective tissue papillae gradually increases.
   (4) Disappearance of hair follicles and sebaceous and sweat glands.
   (5) Disappearance of pigmentation.
   (6) Appearance of labial (seromucous) glands in the connective tissue beneath the oral mucosa.

B. Lining of the Mouth (Oral) Cavity

1. MUCOSA (MUCOUS MEMBRANE)

a. EPITHELIUM. It is stratified squamous. Its thickness varies in different parts of the oral cavity.

b. LAMINA (TUNICA) PROPRIA. It consists chiefly of fine areolar tissue which is thrown into papillae. It blends in most parts of the mouth with a submucosal layer.

2. SUBMUCOSA. This is composed of firm areolar tissue.

3. TISSUES BENEATH THE SUBMUCOSA. These vary in different parts of the mouth. In the cheeks, for example, the mucosa and submucosa lie against muscle. On the other hand, in the hard palate, the lamina propria lies directly against bone.

4. GLANDS. They are small branched structures present almost everywhere in the mouth except in the gums and hard palate.
They contribute to the formation of saliva.

a. MUCOUS GLANDS. These are light-staining in ordinary hematoxylin-eosin preparations. The secretion is thick and slimy. Nuclei may be compressed to the base of cell filled with mucus.

b. SEROUS (ALBUMINOUS) GLANDS. Stain more deeply than mucous glands with hematoxylin-eosin; therefore, they are darker. They produce a watery fluid.

c. MIXED (SEROMUCOUS) GLANDS. The relative number of mucous to serous cells varies considerably.

C. Tongue

1. MUCOSA (MUCOUS MEMBRANE)

a. EPITHELIUM. Thick layer of stratified squamous.

(1) Lingual Papillae. The upper surface of the tongue is studded with projections known as lingual papillae.

(a) Filiform papillae. These are the most numerous of the lingual papillae and are distributed over the entire dorsal surface of the tongue. Each consists of a long slender core of connective tissue covered by epithelium.

(b) Fungiform. They are so named because each somewhat resembles a mushroom. These are unevenly distributed among the filiform papillae. They may contain some taste buds.

(c) Circumvallate (vallate) papillae. These are the largest papillae. The epithelium is not keratinized and contains taste buds. Vallate papillae are grouped along a V-shaped line on the posterior surface of the dorsum of the tongue. They are similar to the fungiform

papillae in outline, but are larger and surrounded by a deep furrow, or valley, from which they derive their name. The serous glands (of von Ebner) open at the bottom of the furrow. Other glands (mucous or mixed) also occur.

(d) Foliate papillae. These are well developed on the tongue of certain rodents such as the rabbit, but are rudimentary in man. In some animals they are parallel folds like the pages (folios) of a book, hence the name foliate. The foliate papillae are not intermingled with the filiform papillae, but occur in groups along the lateral margin of the posterior part of the tongue. They have numerous well-developed taste buds.

2. **LAMINA (TUNICA) PROPRIA.** It is composed of connective tissue, which forms the core of the papillae.

3. **SUBMUCOSA.** Not present on the upper surface of the tongue, where the lamina propria unites directly with the connective tissue of the underlying muscle.

4. **MUSCULATURE.** The tongue can be easily identified by the unique character of the complex musculature. *Although the bundles of striated fibers interlace in all directions, three fairly distinct planes —vertical, transverse, and longitudinal—can be differentiated.* The bundles of muscle fibers are embedded in fibroelastic tissue and variable amounts of fat cells. Seromucous glands sometimes occur among the muscle bundles.

D. Teeth

1. **GENERAL CONSIDERATIONS.** A tooth consists of a crown covered by enamel and a root or roots implanted within the socket. The tooth is composed of enamel, dentin, and cementum, which are calcified tissue. In addition, each tooth has a vascular connective tissue component, known as the pulp and located within the pulp cavity. This cavity extends throughout the root as the root canal, and into part of the crown as the pulp chamber. Hardness of the tooth makes it impossible to prepare sections in the usual manner. Two types of sections of tooth may be prepared: (1) ground sections and (2) decalcified sections. However, only ground sections of mature enamel can be prepared.

2. **ENAMEL.** Enamel is the hardest calcified tissue in the body. Chemically it is 96% inorganic material and 4% organic substance and water. Enamel is composed of slender enamel rods or prisms covered by rod sheaths and a cementing interprismatic substance.

3. **DENTIN.** It is somewhat harder than bone, which it resembles in structure; however, it lacks cells and blood vessels. Chemically,

dentin is 70% inorganic material and 30% organic matter and water. It constitutes the bulk of the tooth and consists of a calcified ground substance, dentinal canals or tubules, and Tomes' dentinal fibrils.

    a. CALCIFIED GROUND SUBSTANCE. Mature dentin is made up of a calcified component called apatite, and an organic component of fine collagenous fibrils arranged in bundles.

    b. DENTINAL CANALS. These begin at the dental pulp and extend outward radially to the periphery of the dentin. In the living state these tubules contain Tomes' dentinal fibrils. The tubules are arranged in the shape of a letter "S" in the crown.

    c. TOMES' DENTINAL FIBRILS. These are protoplasmic processes of the odontoblasts which originate in the pulp.

4. CEMENTUM. Cementum forms a thin shell around the periphery of the root. It is composed of fibrillated, interstitial bone substance. Near the apex, bone cells (cementocytes) are imbedded in thickness with age, the Haversian systems with blood vessels are normally absent. However, as the layer of cementum increases in thickness with age, the Haversian systems with blood vessels may appear. Coarse collagenous bundles from the periodontal membrane penetrate the cementum. These fibers of Sharpey are uncalcified, and in ground sections of the macerated tooth appear as empty canals.

5. PERIODONTAL (PERIDENTAL) MEMBRANE. This is the connective tissue which surrounds the root of the tooth and anchors it to the bony alveolus, attaches the teeth to each other, supports the free margin of the gingiva, and holds it to the tooth. The periodontal membrane is composed of fibrous tissue, fibroblasts, cementoblasts, osteoblasts, blood vessels, and nerves.

6. DENTAL PULP. It fills the pulp cavity which consists of the coronal pulp chamber and the root canals.

    a. PULP TISSUE. It consists of a vascular connective tissue and sensory nerve tissue. The ground substance is soft, gelatinous, and basophilic. It contains numerous thin collagenous fibrils which are not combined into bundles but run in every direction. The pulp cells are similar to those of fibroblasts.

    b. ODONTOBLASTS. These are large, long, peripheral cells, with processes which pass into the dentinal canals. The odontoblasts produce dentin; therefore, they are comparable with osteoblasts.

E. Palate

1. HARD. Bony roof over the mouth. It is lined on its under surface by a mucous membrane. The layers from without inward are:

    a. Stratified squamous epithelium with cornified surface cells.

    b. Lamina propria, continuous with the periosteum of the bone above.

2. SOFT. Continues posteriorly from the hard palate. It is formed by mucous membranes on two sides of a layer of tissue composed of skeletal muscle, fibrous connective tissue, and glands. It is suspended from the hard palate in the manner of a curtain, acting as a partial partition between the mouth and pharynx. Hence the mucous membrane on its upper surface forms the lining of the nasopharynx, and the mucous membrane on its lower surface forms part of the lining of the oral pharynx. From the nasal surface to the oral surface, it exhibits the following layers:

    a. Stratified squamous or pseudostratified ciliated columnar epithelium.

    b. Lamina propria containing few glands.

    c. Striated muscle layer.

    d. Thick lamina propria containing many glands.

    e. Stratified squamous epithelium.

F. Pharynx

1. Epithelium. Upper portion (nasopharynx) may be covered with stratified squamous or pseudostratified ciliated columnar epithelium. Lower portion (oropharynx) lined with stratified squamous epithelium.
2. Lamina Propria. Consists of dense connective tissue.
3. *Muscularis mucosae absent, but an elastic layer instead.*
4. *Striated voluntary muscle not in definite layers.*
5. Mucous or seromucous glands may penetrate the muscle layer.
6. Lymphatic tissue present.

G. Esophagus

1. *Usually in a characteristically collapsed condition, and exhibits a flattened or stellate lumen.*
   a. Mucosa
      (1) *Thick stratified squamous epithelium.* Papillated lower border.
      (2) Lamina propria narrow, solitary lymphatic nodules.
      (3) Muscularis mucosae begins near cricoid cartilage and attains greatest thickness near the stomach.
2. Submucosa consists of thick collagenous and coarse elastic fibers.
3. Muscularis (muscularis externa).
   a. Muscle is in two definite layers with nerve plexus (Auerbach's) between.

b. Muscle is all striated in upper third, mixed in middle third, and nearly all smooth in lower third.
4. Glands:
    a. *Esophageal glands, scattered, extending into submucosa* as tubuloalveolar endpieces; secretory portions in man composed only of mucous cells.
    b. *Cardiac glands,* terminal portions are branched. Mucouslike glands only. Found in the upper and lower parts of the esophagus. Similar to the glands in the cardiac portion of the stomach. *Confined to the lamina propria.* Individual variations and sometimes entirely absent.
    c. In some species no glands are found. *Examples:* rodents, cats, horses.
5. The outer coat, tunica adventitia, consists of loose fibroelastic tissue. The peritoneal lining covers that portion of the esophagus which extends below the diaphragm.

H. Gastroesophageal Junction

1. A longitudinal section through the esophagus at its junction with the stomach shows the following structural characteristics:
    a. Abrupt change from stratified squamous to simple columnar epithelium.
    b. The mucosa increases in thickness in making the transition. The muscularis mucosae is continuous across the junction, as are also the submucosa and muscle layers.
    c. The circular muscle layer increases in thickness to form the cardiac sphincter at the point where the esophagus joins the stomach.

I. Stomach

1. GENERAL STRUCTURE OF STOMACH WALL
    a. Mucosa
        (1) Epithelium. Consists of a single columnar layer of cells which have a length two to four times their width, and rests on a basement membrane.
        (2) Lamina (Tunica) Propria. Consists of collagenous and argyrophilic fibrils and is almost devoid of elastic elements. Meshes of fibers contain pale oval nuclei, small lymphocytes, some plasma cells, eosinophil leukocytes, and mast cells.
        (3) Muscularis Mucosae. Composed of an inner circular and an outer longitudinal layer of smooth muscle; in some places there is a third outer circular layer.

(4) No villi but mucosa folded into ridges or rugae when stomach is not distended.

b. SUBMUCOSA. Consists of a layer of areolar tissue, serving to unite the mucous membrane loosely to the muscularis. The submucosa supports blood vessels, lymphatics, and the submucous (Meissner's) nerve plexus.

c. MUSCULARIS (MUSCULARIS EXTERNA). Usually described as consisting of three layers, but in the fundus, muscle fibers run in various directions. The demonstration of the muscle layers in sections is somewhat difficult.

(1) Inner oblique layer of muscle.

(2) Middle circular layer of muscle.

(3) Outer, mainly, longitudinal layer of muscle.

d. SEROSA

(1) Inner layer of loose connective tissue attached to the muscularis externa.

(2) Outer covering of mesothelium.

2. SPECIFIC REGIONS OF STOMACH

a. CARDIAC

(1) Simple columnar epithelium.

(2) *Goblet cells are absent in all parts of the stomach as contrasted with the intestine;* there may be very rare exceptions to this statement.

(3) No gastric glands extend into submucosa.

(4) *Cardiac glands of the stomach,* according to Bensley, occupy only a limited area adjacent to the esophagus.

(5) *Scattered parietal cells may be found in the cardiac region.*

b. FUNDUS

(1) Gastric (principal) glands occupy a much larger area than the fundus.

(a) *Gastric pits extend down into the mucosa less than one-half its thickness.*

(b) *Dark-staining gastric glands abundant in the mucosa, with many eosinophilic parietal cells.*

(c) *Glands shorter but more branched than in the cardiac stomach.*

(d) Gland tubule consists of neck, body, and fundus. The lumen is so narrow as to be almost imperceptible, and the effect produced is that of a cord of cells.

(*1*) Mucous neck cells.

(*2*) *Chief (zymogenic) cells:* columnar, squarish or wedge-shaped predominate; *bluish-staining,* and granular.

(*3*) *Parietal (oxyntic) cells:* large, clear, and *eosinophilic (pink).*

c. PYLORUS

   (1) *Gastric pits extend down into the mucosa more than one-half its thickness.*

   (2) *Light-staining pyloric glands,* consisting of mucouslike cells above muscularis mucosae and *with very deep pits.*

   (3) *The glands are of the simple branched type, but the divisions are more numerous, the lumen is larger, and the tubules more coiled than in the fundus.* Therefore, in perpendicular sections they are seldom seen as longitudinal structures.

   (4) Few parietal cells, only near pyloric sphincter and the fundic border.

   (5) Solitary lymph nodules in cardiac and in pyloric portions of stomach.

3. GENERAL CONSIDERATIONS

   a. Cardiac, fundic, and pyloric regions are not separated by sharply drawn limits.

   b. Along the border lines of these regions the glands of one region mix with those of the other.

J. Small Intestine

1. GENERAL STRUCTURE OF INTESTINAL WALL
The layers from within outward are:

   a. MUCOSA

      (1) Epithelium.

      (2) Lamina (Tunica) Propria.

      (3) Muscularis Mucosae.

         (a) Inner circular layer of smooth muscle.

         (b) Outer longitudinal layer of smooth muscle.

   b. SUBMUCOSA

      (1) Dense connective tissue with numerous elastic networks. Occasional lobules of adipose tissue.

      (2) In duodenum it is occupied by duodenal glands.

   c. MUSCULARIS

      (1) Thick inner circular layer of smooth muscle.

      (2) Thinner outer longitudinal layer of smooth muscle.

   d. SEROSA (TUNICA SEROSA)

      (1) Loose connective tissue covered by a layer of mesothelium.

2. SPECIFIC STRUCTURES OF INTESTINAL WALL

   a. VILLI

      (1) *Fingerlike projections of mucosa, surrounded by simple columnar epithelium with striated (cuticular) border.*

      (2) When sectioned, portions of the villi may appear as islands of connective tissue surrounded by epithelium.

b. GLANDS OF LIEBERKÜHN (CRYPTS OF LIEBERKÜHN OR INTESTINAL GLANDS)

(1) Located at base of villi.

(2) When cross-sectioned, crypts appear as holes in the connective tissue lined with simple columnar epithelium.

c. PANETH CELLS

(1) Large pink-staining or clear sharp-edged eosinophilic granules are found in the cell cytoplasm at the bottom of the glands of Lieberkühn. Not found in dogs.

d. ARGENTAFFINE CELLS

(1) These cells have been demonstrated in all parts of the alimentary tract, from the esophagus to the anus, but are most numerous in small intestine, therefore mentioned here.

(2) Their cytoplasm contains argyrophilic granules. These cells are located between the cells lining the glands of Lieberkühn.

e. GOBLET CELLS

(1) More numerous as one approaches colon.

3. **SPECIFIC REGIONS OF SMALL INTESTINE**

a. DUODENUM

(1) *Brunner's (duodenal) glands in the submucosa.* Presence of Brunner's glands in the upper duodenum is an identifying feature, but in the lower part of the duodenum these glands are absent. Gland cells stain like mucous cells.

(2) *Villi are low, broad, leaflike,* with glands of Lieberkühn at their bases which extend to the muscularis mucosae but do not penetrate it.

(3) If the *bile duct or ampulla of Vater* shows in the wall, it is duodenum.

(4) Serosa covers exposed surface only.

b. JEJUNUM

(1) *Villi taller and more slender with a more extensive development of the plicae circulares than in the duodenum.*

(2) More goblet cells than in the duodenum.

(3) *Solitary nodules do not extend into the submucosa.*

c. ILEUM

(1) *Few, short, club-shaped villi and scattered plicae.*

(2) *Greater accumulations of lymphatic tissue than in jejunum.*

(3) *Peyer's patches are to be found in the portion of the wall opposite the attachment of the mesentery.* They consist of flask-shaped lymphatic nodules. The epithelium covering the area above the nodules is greatly reduced, and the villi are short or entirely absent.

(4) More goblet cells than in the jejunum.

(5) Nerves.
(a) Myenteric (Auerbach's) plexus, located between circular and longitudinal muscles.
(b) Submucous (Meissner's) plexus, located in the submucosa.

K. Large Intestine

1. SPECIFIC REGIONS

a. COLON

(1) *Mucosa relatively smooth as compared with that of the stomach or small intestine. No villi. Tubular pits or glands present.* Lined with simple columnar epithelium.

(2) *More goblet cells than in small intestine.*

(3) Simple tubular glands, longer than those of small intestine; but, if cross-sectioned, are of about the same size at top and bottom.

(4) Paneth cells usually absent.

(5) *Solitary nodules of lymphatic tissue numerous.*

(6) *Outer longitudinal muscle layer is massed in three thick bands, the taeniae (lineae) coli. In a given section the longitudinal muscle layer may be thick or thin depending on the presence or absence of the taeniae coli.*

(7) Serosa contains lobules of fat which form pendulous projections, called appendices epiploicae.

b. CECUM (CAECUM)

(1) Structure is similar to that of the colon; usually there is more lymphatic tissue than in the colon but less than in the appendix.

c. VERMIFORM APPENDIX

(1) Lumen which varies in size and shape is thrown into deep and pocketed folds.

(2) Lumen, frequently, totally occluded as result of fibrosis in adult; however, if lumen present:
(a) Tends to be small and cleftlike in cross section.
(b) Lumen changes with age from being three-horned in youth to circular, slitlike, and other shapes in the adult.
(c) *Fecal concretions frequently found in lumen.*

(3) Wall of appendix relatively thick.

(4) *No pits or villi.*

(5) *Large amount of lymphatic tissue which may extend into the submucosa.*

(6) Glands of Lieberkühn more frequently branched than in colon.

(7) Usually little or no distinct muscularis mucosae because it is crowded out by lymphatic nodules.

(8) Inner circular and outer longitudinal muscle layers, but longitudinal layer differs from that of the large intestine in not being arranged into taeniae; in other words, the taeniae coli are absent.

(9) The appendix is composed of the same tissue elements as those which form the colon, but in the appendix the glands are less numerous and there is much more lymphatic tissue.

d. RECTUM

(1) *The glands of Lieberkühn are longer and contain a wider lumen than those of the colon.*

(2) *Goblet cells are present in such numbers that they form by far the greater portion of the epithelial lining of the crypts.*

(3) The longitudinal muscle of the taeniae coli spreads out in the rectum to form a continuous coat of uniform thickness; however, it may be thickened on one or two sides.

e. ANAL CANAL

(1) *Longitudinal sections in the lower portion show a transition from simple columnar to stratified columnar, and finally to stratified squamous epithelium* which is continuous with the skin in much the same fashion as the lip.

(2) Lower cutaneous portion may be confused with the lip.

(3) The skin may be identified by the hairs associated with it.

(4) Near anal opening are *circumanal glands* (similar to sweat glands).

(5) Circular layer of the muscularis coat is thickened around the anus to form two sphincters; the upper one of these is composed of smooth muscle, but the lower one consists of striated muscle.

TABLE 7. SUMMARY OF THE HISTOLOGY OF THE DIGESTIVE SYSTEM*

Organ	Epithelium	Muscularis Mucosae	Muscle Layers	Lymphatic Tissue	Glands			
					Name and Type	Position	Kinds of Cells	
Pharynx	Upper portion, stratified squamous, stratified columnar, or pseudostratified ciliated. Lower portion, stratified squamous	Elastic layers instead of muscle	Striated voluntary muscle, not in two definite layers	Pharyngeal and palatine tonsils. Nodules and diffuse areas	Pharyngeal, simple branched, tubuloalveolar	Extend down into connective tissue and down into the edge of muscle	Mucous and seromucous	
Esophagus	Stratified squamous	Consists of longitudinal smooth muscle fibers and thin elastic network	Two layers. Upper third, inner circular and outer longitudinal striated muscle Middle third, circular and longitudinal striated and smooth muscle Lower third, circular and longitudinal smooth muscle. Exception in man where striated fibers are found even at cardiac orifice	Relatively few nodules in man; diffuse	Esophageal: mucous glands. Branching tubuloalveolar glands. Seromucous glands in some lower mammals. Cardiac in lower portion.	Extend into mucosa and submucosa	Mucous cells only in man. In some lower mammals mucous and serous occur	

*Lamina (tunica) propria and submucosa omitted because of space limitations.

144

Organ	Epithelium	Muscularis Mucosae	Muscle Layers	Lymphatic Tissue	Glands Name and Type	Glands Position	Glands Kinds of Cells
Cardiac	Simple columnar	Inner circular and outer longitudinal, and in some places a third outer circular layer of smooth muscle	Inner oblique, middle circular, and outer longitudinal layers of smooth muscle. Oblique layer not distinguishable in some places	Small areas of lymphatic tissue in lamina propria adjacent to muscularis mucosae. Some may extend into submucosa	Cardiac	Lamina propria and some may extend into submucosa	Mucous and occasional parietal cells
Fundus	Simple columnar	Same as cardiac stomach	Myenteric (Auerbach's) plexus between circular and longitudinal muscle layers	Same as cardiac stomach	Gastric glands are simple branched tubular glands with short pits and long secreting pockets	Same as cardiac stomach	Chief cells. Parietal cells. Mucous cells
Pyloris	Simple columnar	Same as cardiac stomach	Myenteric (Auerbach's) plexus between circular and longitudinal muscle layers	Small nodules in lamina propria	Pyloric glands, chiefly simple branched tubular glands with deep pits and short secreting pockets	Same as cardiac stomach	Pale and mucouslike. Occasional parietal cells

Stomach

145

TABLE 7. SUMMARY OF THE HISTOLOGY OF THE DIGESTIVE SYSTEM* (Continued)

Organ	Epithelium	Muscularis Mucosae	Muscle Layers	Lymphatic Tissue	Glands Name and Type	Glands Position	Kinds of Cells
Duodenum	Simple columnar	Inner circular and outer longitudinal layers of smooth muscle	Inner circular. Outer longitudinal layers of smooth muscle. Myenteric (Auerbach's) plexus between circular and longitudinal muscle	Solitary nodules and diffuse areas	1. Duodenal (Brunner's) glands: compound tubular glands of mucous type 2. Glands of Lieberkühn	Brunner's glands, chiefly in submucosa. Glands of Lieberkühn above muscularis mucosae	1. Paneth cells, large cells in epithelium which lines distal portions of crypts. Characterized by eosinophilic granules 2. Mucouslike cells of Brunner's glands 3. Cells of glands of Lieberkühn 4. Goblet cells 5. Argentaffin cells between cells of glands of Lieberkühn
Jejunum	Simple columnar	Same as duodenum	Same as duodenum	Same as duodenum	Glands of Lieberkühn: simple tubular glands above muscularis mucosae	In small intestine and in large intestine above muscularis mucosae	Same as duodenum. Small and large intestines possess goblet cells which increase relatively from upper to lower part of intestine

Small Intestine

* Lamina (tunica) propria and submucosa omitted because of space limitations.

| | | | | | Glands | | |
Organ	Epithelium	Muscularis Mucosae	Muscle Layers	Lymphatic Tissue	Name and Type	Position	Kinds of Cells
Ileum	Simple columnar	Same as duodenum	Same as duodenum	Aggregate (Peyer's) nodules and diffuse areas	Same as jejunum	Same as jejunum	Same as duodenum
Colon	Simple columnar	Same as duodenum	An internal circular layer of smooth muscle is typical. An external layer of three longitudinal strands of smooth muscle (taeniae coli).	Solitary nodules and diffuse areas	Same as jejunum	Same as jejunum	Same as duodenum, except absence of cells of Paneth
Rectum	Simple columnar	Same as duodenum	Inner circular and outer longitudinal layers of smooth muscle	Solitary nodules	Crypts longer with wider lumen than those of jejunum	Same as jejunum	Increased number of goblet cells
Anal Canal	Upper part, simple columnar which changes to stratified columnar, and finally stratified squamous in lower portion	Spreads out fanlike in rectal columns (columns of Morgagni) and forms the dilator muscle of Rudinger	Varies as to the region. Upper part smooth; near anus striated	Solitary nodules in submucosa	Lower portion sebaceous. Near anal openings, circumanal (similar to sweat glands)	Varies with type of gland	Mucous and other types peculiar to different glands

Large Intestine

147

Chapter 14   GLANDS OF THE DIGESTIVE SYSTEM

A. Salivary Glands

1. PAROTID

a. *In adults, a purely serous (albuminous) gland.*

b. *Intercalated (intralobular) ducts lined with low cuboidal or flat epithelium.*

c. Secretory (intralobular) ducts lined with simple columnar epithelium. Their basal portions have a characteristic striated appearance.

d. *No islands or centroacinous cells (see pancreas).*

e. The general structure is like that of the pancreas, but there are several marked differences: the parotid has many more ducts than the pancreas and it possesses no islands of Langerhans or centroacinous cells. Parenchyma of parotid stains darker with hematoxylin than pancreas.

f. Groups of fat cells in the connective tissue are characteristic of parotid gland.

2. SUBMAXILLARY (SUBMANDIBULAR)

a. Most of the secretory endpieces are serous alveoli, rounded to somewhat elongate.

b. Mixed serous and mucous cells (see p. 34 for description), with serous predominating; *about four-fifths serous, one-fifth mucous* in man. In cat and dog the submaxillary gland resembles the sublingual.

c. *Most of the mucous alveoli (acini) are capped by serous demilunes.*

d. *Intercalated (intralobular) ducts present.*

e. *Secretory salivary (intralobular) ducts usually longer than in sublingual.*

3. SUBLINGUAL

a. *Mixed serous and mucous cells, with at least one-half mucous in man.*

   b. Chiefly mucous alveoli, but some serous demilunes.
   c. *The slender intercalated ducts may be absent.*
   d. *Lymphoid tissue may be scattered through gland, especially in the connective tissue septa.*
   e. Connective tissue septa are usually more prominent than in the parotid or submaxillary glands.
   f. Connective tissue capsule not nearly so definite as in the parotid and submaxillary glands.
4. **ORAL (BUCCAL) AND LABIAL**
   a. Seromucous, serous, and mucous alveoli.
5. **PALATINE**
   a. Mucous cells only.
6. **ANTERIOR LINGUAL GLAND**
   a. Posterior part of gland of mucous and seromucous cells.
   b. Anterior part of gland, seromucous cells only.
   c. Generally shows some tongue muscle under and between the areas of gland tissue.
7. **POSTERIOR LINGUAL GLANDS (OF VON EBNER)**
   a. Serous cells only. Rarely mixed.
   b. A section often shows stratified squamous epithelium and tongue muscle.

B. Pancreas

1. Superficially resembles the salivary glands, especially the parotid, in structure.
2. *Spheroidal aggregations of light-staining cells, islets of Langerhans, usually found interposed among pancreatic acini.* They are the most distinctive feature in the pancreas since they persist when the secretory acini have entirely disappeared as the result of a pancreatic pathology. May be absent in head of pancreas.
3. *Centroacinous cells are present in the pancreatic acini.*
4. Zymogen granules may often be observed in the cytoplasm of the cells of the acini.
5. Note the two-zone staining effect in acinar cells: the apex stains acidic and the basal cell half stains more basic.
6. *Interlobular connective tissue greater in amount and looser than in parotid.*
7. *Few ducts, two to five, under medium power (100 diameters) field.*
8. No intralobular secretory ducts.

C. Liver

1. *Lobules indefinite* in man, about two-thirds the size of medium power (100 diameters) field. Lobules definite in pig.

2. *Central vein* is the center of the lobule in man.
3. *Portal canal* (*islands of Glisson; trinity*), located at periphery of lobule; consisting of a little connective tissue, containing the *portal vein, hepatic artery,* and one or more *bile ducts.*
4. Hepatic cells are large polygonal cells with one or two eccentric, deeply staining, spherical nuclei.
5. Elias described the parenchyma of the human liver as being arranged in the form of perforated anastomosing plates. These enclose spaces in which sinusoids are present, and the sinusoids communicate with each other through perforations in the plates.
6. According to the Elias concept, it is the plates of liver cells which have been conventionally described as liver "cords."
7. Bile canaliculi within the anastomosing perforated plates of parenchyma form a very complicated branching network.

D. Gallbladder

1. Epithelium is simple columnar; *ovoid nuclei near base; peripheral part large and clear. No goblet cells.*
2. *Mucous membrane is raised in a series of folds.* The tall primary folds give rise to secondary folds which unite with one another and enclose pockets of varying size. The pseudoglandular structures which result may extend well out into the muscular wall.
3. *Muscular wall is very unusual in that smooth muscle is interspersed with connective tissue. The muscles are arranged in small pencil-like bundles which are separated by connective tissue.*
4. *Entire wall is thin compared with the intestine.*

E. Common Bile Duct

1. *Epithelium consists mainly of tall columnar cells, resmbling cells of the gallbladder, but is unlike the gallbladder epithelium in that goblet cells are found here and there in the epithelium.*
2. Branched, tubular, mucus-secreting glands in the subepithelial layer.

Chapter 15   RESPIRATORY SYSTEM

The respiratory system consists of the nasal cavities, pharynx, larynx, trachea, bronchi, and bronchioles. In the bronchial tubes there is a gradual change from thick-walled rigid structures to thinner and softer tubules, a change somewhat like that occurring in the blood vessels.

A. Nasal Cavity

1. **VESTIBULE**
   a. Lined with stratified squamous epithelium continuous with the skin of the nose.
2. **OLFACTORY REGION** (described in detail on p. 218).
3. **RESPIRATORY REGION**
   a. Pseudostratified ciliated columnar epithelium.
   b. The subepithelial connective tissue is not differentiated into a distinct lamina propria and submucosa. Seromucous glands present.

B. Nasopharynx

1. The nasopharynx is lined with either pseudostratified or stratified epithelium, regionally.

C. Pharynx

1. Inspired air crosses the pharynx. See description on p. 130.

D. Larynx

1. *Epithelium chiefly pseudostratified ciliated columnar; but where the surface is exposed to friction or abrasion, as over the true vocal cords and epiglottis, stratified squamous is found.* At junction of these two types, stratified ciliated columnar may be present.
2. There is a definite basement membrane but *no muscularis mucosae*. There is no sharp demarcation between the mucosa and submucosa.
3. Cartilages of the larynx are: epiglottis, thyroid, cricoid, cuneiform,

corniculate, and arytenoids; the latter three appear in pairs. The cartilages are usually hyaline with the exception of the epiglottis, cuneiform, corniculate, and parts of the arytenoids in which yellow elastic tissue occurs.

4. There are two sets of muscles, extrinsic and intrinsic. The extrinsic muscles connect various parts of the larynx with surrounding muscles and tissues. The intrinsic muscles run between different cartilages of the larynx.

5. True vocal cords have striated muscle; false vocal cords are muscleless.

6. *Mucous and seromucous glands.*

E. Trachea

1. *Chiefly pseudostratified ciliated columnar epithelium.* Numerous goblet cells scattered through the epithelium.

2. Broad basement membrane.

3. Lamina propria contains a layer of reticular fibers.

4. At the outer border of the lamina propria, in a position comparable to the muscularis mucosae in the intestine, is an elastic membrane of coarse fibers.

5. Submucosa in which tracheal glands are composed of mucous and serous cells.

6. *Supported by incomplete rings of hyaline cartilage, either ovoid in cross section, or long pieces in longitudinal section.*

7. The posterior part of the trachea has no cartilage but has considerable smooth muscle (trachealis), which connects the free ends of the semilunar (C-shaped) cartilages. Longitudinal fasciculi of muscle may be present although the muscle bundles run transversely for the most part.

8. Connective tissue is present between the rings of cartilage and in the outer wall.

F. Bronchi

1. Primary bronchi have the same structure as the trachea, but in their subdivisions changes occur as follows:

   a. Epithelium, although continuing as pseudostratified columnar type, decreases in height as the tubes become progressively smaller.

   b. *C-shaped cartilaginous ring is replaced by irregular plates of cartilage which may completely surround the bronchus.*

2. Mucosa appears wavy in cross section because of the longitudinal folding due to the contraction of muscle.

3. Seromucous glands are in the submucosa, especially between the cartilages, and may spread out below them.

4. Some smooth muscle between the ends of cartilages; the amount of cartilage decreases as the amount of muscle increases.

5. *May have lung tissue or lymphatic nodules in a section.*

G. Bronchioles

1. The ciliated epithelium varies from columnar to cuboidal as the tubes become smaller. In the smallest respiratory bronchioles the cubical cells are not ciliated.

2. The mucosa of the terminal bronchioles is folded longitudinally. *The mucosa shows marked waviness in cross section.*

3. *Cartilage disappears when the diameter of the bronchiole reaches 1 mm in diameter.* The glands also are absent but goblet cells still occur.

4. Two major points to remember in regard to bronchioles are:
   a. Muscle is the main element of the wall.
   b. Cilia persist more distally than mucous cells.

H. Lung

1. Alveolar ducts can be identified as communicating spaces whose walls are closely beset with thin-walled outpocketings, the alveolar (air) sacs. The intervening portions consist of strands of collagenous and elastic fibers and smooth muscle cells.

   It has been demonstrated by electron microscope studies that each alveolus is lined with a simple squamous epithelium.

   In tissues which have lost all nuclear staining power, lung alveoli can be recognized by the fact that the ultimate alveolar spaces are separated in part from one another by incomplete septa. *This is the only place in the body in which incomplete septa can be found in a structure of this general pattern.*

2. *May contain bronchi or bronchioles.*

3. Many conspicuous black particles of carbon may be present in the cytoplasm of dust cells (alveolar phagocytes).

4. Visceral layer of the pleura envelops the lung. The surface of the pleura is covered with a mesothelium which rests upon a sub-mesothelial layer of connective tissue.

5. Lymphatic tissue may or may not be prominent.

TABLE 8. SUMMARY OF THE HISTOLOGY OF THE RESPIRATORY SYSTEM

Organ	Epithelium	Lamina Propria	Muscle Layers	Glands		
				Name and Type	Position	Kinds of Cells
Vestibule	Stratified squamous	Collagenous and elastic fibers with papillae	None	Sebaceous and sweat glands	Subepithelial connective tissue	Sebaceous and sweat gland cells
Olfactory Region	Pseudostratified	Collagenous and elastic fibers; in deep portion blends with periosteum	None	Olfactory (Bowman's) glands. Branched tubular	Stroma	Serous
Respiratory Region	Pseudostratified ciliated. On conchae, varies from simple columnar on under surface to pseudostratified and even stratified squamous on upper surface	Collagenous and elastic fibers; toward bone merge with periosteum. Very vascular	None	Branched tubular	Subepithelial connective tissue	Goblet cells. Mucous and serous
Pharynx	Upper portion, stratified squamous, or pseudostratified ciliated columnar. Lower portion stratified squamous	Collagenous and elastic fibers. Contains many lymphocytes and nodules (pharyngeal tonsil)	Striated voluntary muscle, not in two definite layers	Pharyngeal, simple branched, tubuloalveolar. Mucous and seromucous glands	Extends down into connective tissue and edge of muscle	Mucous and seromucous
Larynx	For most part pseudostratified ciliated columnar. Where friction or abrasion, stratified squamous as over true vocal cords and epiglottis	Collagenous and elastic fibers. Lymphocytes and solitary nodules present. Whole layer much reduced	Extrinsic muscles, intrinsic muscles, muscles associated with true vocal cords	Branched tubular	Stroma, and may extend down into intermuscular connective tissue	Mucous and serous

Nasal

Tube

es

Organ	Epithelium	Lamina Propria	Muscle Layers	Glands		
				Name and Type	Position	Kinds of Cells
Trachea	Chiefly pseudostratified ciliated columnar	Collagenous, reticular, and many elastic fibers. Lymphatic tissue diffuse and in the form of nodules	Between free ends of cartilage, smooth muscle (trachealis)	Tracheal glands, simple, branched, usually present	Chiefly submucosa	Goblet cells. Mucous and serous
Bronchi	Pseudostratified ciliated columnar	Collagenous and elastic fibers. Lymphocytes present. Entire layer reduced	Smooth circular muscle. In primary bronchi same as trachea	Bronchial glands, branched tublar	Usually between cartilages	Same as trachea
Bronchioles	Ciliated or nonciliated, columnar or cuboidal	Further reduced. Collagenous and elastic fibers	Smooth circular muscle	None	None	None
Respiratory Bronchioles	Low columnar, cuboidal, or squamous	Collagenous and elastic fibers	Smooth muscle fibers	None	None	None
Alveolar Ducts	Squamous	Collagenous and elastic fibers	Strands of smooth muscle fibers	None	None	None
Alveoli (Air Sacs)	Simple squamous	Elastic and reticular fibers	None	None	None	None

Tubes

Lung

Chapter 16   URINARY SYSTEM

A. Kidney

1. CORTEX

a. Thin, eosinophilic, connective tissue capsule on surface.

b. *Renal corpuscles distinctly blue when stained with H. and E. Generally appear as rounded cellular masses.*

c. *Labyrinth (pars convoluta), a mass of convoluted tubules between renal corpuscles.*

    (1) Proximal convoluted tubules 60 microns in diameter. Cells are truncated pyramidal in form and *usually stain deeply with eosin. Free surface of cells possesses a brush border.* The brush border is seldom seen in routine preparations because it undergoes rapid postmortem changes. Cell boundaries are rarely seen.

    (2) Distal convoluted tubules 20–50 microns in diameter. *Distinguished from proximal convoluted tubules in that the cells are lower, more cuboidal, smaller, stain less deeply with eosin, show fainter basal striations, and show no brush border.* Cell boundaries are fairly distinct.

d. Medullary rays may show with very low power.

2. MEDULLA

a. *A solid mass of cross-sectioned or longitudinally sectioned tubules of three sizes:*

    (1) Henle's loop:

        (a) Descending limb is about 14–22 microns in diameter. Thick part like proximal convoluted tubule. Thin segment composed of squamous epithelial cells with pale-staining cytoplasm. Thin segment may be mistaken for a capillary.

        (b) Ascending limb is about 33 microns in diameter. Thick part is lined with simple cuboidal epithelium.

    (2) Collecting tubules vary in diameter from 40–200 microns with large lumen; upper portion, cuboidal epithelium; lower portion, columnar epithelium. *The epithelium lining all parts of the collecting tubules has a faintly staining cytoplasm, round dark-staining nuclei, and distinct cell membranes.*

3. PELVIS

a. Mucosa (mucous membrane).
  (1) Lined with transitional epithelium, three to four cells in thickness
  (2) Lamina propria thin.
b. Muscularis (muscular coat). Smooth muscle.
c. Adventitia. Loose fibroelastic connective tissue.

B. Ureter

1. MUCOSA (MUCOUS MEMBRANE)

a. *Irregular lumen lined with transitional epithelium.*
b. Lamina (tunica) propria and submucosa usually merge together.
  (1) Delicate white fibers, with which a few elastic fibers are intermingled.
c. Muscularis mucosae absent.
d. In some places a thin layer of smooth muscle fibers appears to divide the connective tissue into a superficial lamina propria and a deeper submucosa.

2. MUSCULARIS (MUSCULAR COAT) consists of coarse smooth muscle bundles with connective tissue among them.

a. Proximal part (upper half).
  (1) *Inner longitudinal layer.*
  (2) *Outer circular layer.*
b. Distal part (lower third).
  (1) Same as proximal except for a third *outer longitudinal muscle layer.*

3. ADVENTITIA (FIBROSA)

a. Loose fibroelastic connective tissue.
b. *Much adipose tissue, often associated with the outer part of adventitia.*

C. Urinary Bladder

1. MUCOSA

a. *Folded Surface.*
  (1) *Transitional epithelium, two-layered in distended bladder and as many as eight layers in the contracted condition.*
  (2) Pits in epithelial surface may be seen which may or may not possess a lumen.
b. *Lamina (Tunica) Propria and Submucosa.*
  (1) These are blended together.
c. *Muscularis mucosae absent.*

2. MUSCULARIS

a. *Rather thick muscular coat* made up of three layers of smooth muscle fibers: outer, longitudinal; middle, circular or spiral; and an innermost layer consisting of separate longitudinal or

oblique strands. Muscle layers cannot be distinctly separated from each other.
3. **SEROSA**
   a. A relatively thick connective tissue layer which is covered in part by mesothelium.

D. Urethra of Female

1. *The lumen is irregularly crescent or U-shaped and usually appears collapsed.*
2. Epithelium.
   a. The epithelium near the bladder is transitional; next come areas of pseudostratified and stratified columnar epithelium; finally near the outlet is stratified squamous epithelium.
3. *Lamina propria, a loose and very vascular connective tissue, constituting the corpus spongiosum.*
4. *Urethral glands usually present.*
5. Paraurethral (Skene's) glands open directly on to the vestibule instead of into the urethra by means of ducts. Not often observed.

E. Urethra of Male

1. **PROSTATIC PART (PARS PROSTATICA)**
   a. Lumen irregular in shape.
   b. Lined by transitional pseudostratified or stratified columnar epithelium.
   c. Lamina propria consists of fibroelastic connective tissue in which are prominent venous spaces.
   d. Muscularis of inner longitudinal and outer circular layers.
   e. *The male prostatic urethra is surrounded more or less by prostate gland tissue.*
2. **MEMBRANOUS PART (PARS MEMBRANACEA)**
   a. *Stratified columnar or pseudostratified epithelium.*
   b. Muscular layers of inner longitudinal and outer circular layers.
   c. Bulbourethral (Cowper's) glands open near the cavernous portion. Their ducts are lined with low epithelium, which is surrounded by thin rings of smooth muscle.
3. **CAVERNOUS PORTION (PARS CAVERNOSUM)**
   a. *Stratified columnar or pseudostratified epithelium.* Patches of stratified squamous epithelium are common.
   b. The urethra shows many glandular outpocketings (lacunae of Morgagni). The outpocketings continue into deeper, branching tubules, the *urethral glands* (Littré's glands).
4. **DISTAL END**
   a. *Epithelium of stratified squamous tissue at the end in the fossa navicularis.*
   b. *Papillae of lamina propria prominent.*

TABLE 9. SUMMARY OF THE HISTOLOGY OF THE URINARY SYSTEM*

	Organ	Epithelium	Lamina (Tunica) Propria	Muscle Layers	Adventitia
	Bowman's Capsule	Flattened	None	None	None
	Proximal Convoluted Tubule	Truncated pyramidal cells with brush border	None	None	None
	Descending Limb of Henle's Loop	Thin segment present, which consists of squamous epithelium	None	None	None
	Ascending Limb of Henle's Loop	Usually thick segment present, which consists of simple cuboidal epithelium	None	None	None
K i d n e y	Distal Convoluted Tubule	Simple cuboidal without brush border. Faint basal striations	None	None	None
	Junctional (Arched) Tubule	Simple cuboidal	None	None	None
	Collecting Tubule	Upper portion, cuboidal. Lower portion, columnar. Variable epithelium	None	None	None
	Papillary Ducts	Simple columnar	None	None	None
	Calyx	Transitional	Elastic and reticular tissue	Inner longitudinal and outer circular layers of smooth muscle	Connective tissue, fibroelastic
	Pelvis	Transitional	Elastic fibers and reticular tissue	Inner longitudinal and outer circular layers of smooth muscle	Fibroelastic tissue

*There is no distinct submucosa in man, but the muscularis mucosae is found in the monkey and in most domestic animals, except the cat.

TABLE 9. SUMMARY OF THE HISTOLOGY OF THE URINARY SYSTEM* (Continued)

	Organ	Epithelium	Lamina (Tunica) Propria	Muscle Layers	Adventitia
	Ureter	Transitional	Collagenous and elastic fibers	Upper portion: inner longitudinal, outer circular. Lower third: inner longitudinal, middle, circular, outer longitudinal	Loose fibroelastic tissue. Adipose tissue present
	Bladder	Transitional	Elastic and reticular tissue	Inner longitudinal or oblique. Middle circular. Outer longitudinal	In nonperitoneal part, fibrous
Urethra	**Urethra (Female)**	Upper portion, transitional. Lower portion, stratified squamous with areas of pseudo-stratified epithelium	Loose connective tissue with elastic fibers. Vascular	Inner longitudinal and outer circular layers of smooth muscle. External sphincter of striated muscle	Fibroelastic tissue
Urethra	**Urethra (Male)**	Prostatic portion: transitional. Membranous portion: stratified columnar, or pseudo-stratified. Cavernous portion: stratified columnar, or pseudo-stratified, patches of stratified squamous. Lower portion: stratified squamous as a rule	Fibroelastic connective tissue	Prostatic and membranous portions: inner longitudinal, outer circular; sphincter muscle of striated fibers	Fibroelastic tissue

* There is no distinct submucosa in man, but the muscularis mucosae is found in the monkey and in most domestic animals, except the cat.

Chapter 17　　　　MALE REPRODUCTIVE SYSTEM

A. Testis (Testicle)

1. Tunica (surrounds testis at periphery).
   a. ALBUGINEA—outer layer consists of densely compacted collagenous and elastic fibers.
   b. VASCULOSA—innermost layer composed of loose connective tissue supporting numerous blood vessels.
   c. CONNECTIVE TISSUE SEPTA extend from tunica albuginea into mediastinum, dividing testis into pyramidal lobules.
2. *Seminiferous (convoluted) tubules* in lobules. In sections, one may get any view of tubules due to their convolutions. *Thus they may appear as ovals, question marks, C's, U's, or S's.* The form of the cut tubule is a valuable identification character.
   a. SEMINIFEROUS EPITHELIUM. From periphery to lumen: spermatogonia, primary spermatocytes, secondary spermatocytes, and spermatids. With the exception of the spermatids, these cells are actively undergoing division and therefore the nuclei stain darkly.
   b. SUSTENTACULAR (SERTOLI) CELLS. Tall cells, irregular in outline, which extend from the basement membrane to the lumen. They support the germinal cells. *The oval nucleus is paler than the nucleus of any of the germinal cells.*
   c. INTERSTITIAL CELLS (CELLS OF LEYDIG).
      (1) Usually occur in dense compact groups of various sizes lying in the stroma of the angular spaces between the tubules.
      (2) Fairly large cells which are ovoid or polygonal in shape. Nucleus is large and often eccentrically located. The cytoplasm stains lightly.
   d. *Spermatozoa may be present in the lumen.*
3. Tubuli recti (straight tubules) are continuous with seminiferous tubules. They are lined with simple epithelial cells which vary from columnar to cuboidal.
4. The tubuli recti pass into the mediastinum, where they empty into

the *rete testis, a branching network of cavernouslike spaces in the mediastinum, lined with cuboidal or squamous epithelium* and surrounded by dense connective tissue.

B. Ductuli (Tubuli) Efferentes

These ductules lead from the rete testis to the epididymis.

1. *Epithelium is unique in that it consists, mainly, of two kinds of cells, groups of tall ciliated cells alternating with short cells which may show secretory blebs.* This type of epithelium makes the lumen *appear scalloped.*
2. *Thin layer of circular smooth muscle. Little muscle as compared with the ductus deferens.*

C. Ductus Epididymis

1. *Lumen of duct lined with an epithelium which consists of a basal layer of small cells and a surface layer of tall columnar cells.* Tall cells and occasionally short ones are stereociliated. Variously classified as *pseudostratified* or stratified columnar.
2. *Tubules with thin fibromuscular walls.*
3. Masses of spermatozoa often found in the lumina of the tubules.
4. *Spaces between tubules filled with a loose connective tissue.*

D. Ductus Deferens (Vas Deferens)

1. *Mucous membrane typically folded in cross section.*
2. Small lumen lined with pseudostratified epithelium which may or may not be stereociliated. The epithelium is lower than in the epididymis; but near the epididymis, the epithelium is like that of the ductus epididymis. Some authors describe the epithelium as columnar nonciliated.
3. *Very thick, dense, muscular wall of interlacing fibers which consists of the following layers: inner and outer longitudinal and middle circular. Inner longitudinal layer poorly developed.* In proportion to the diameter of its lumen the ductus deferens is one of the most muscular tubes in the human body.
4. Generally one to several arteries present outside of muscle, but no large vessels in muscle wall.
5. Adventitia (fibrosa) of connective tissue.

E. Ampulla of Ductus Deferens

1. Epithelium is cuboidal or columnar.
2. Mucosa is thrown into numerous branching folds which in many places fuse with one another, thus in section appearing netlike.
3. *Resembles the seminal vesicles but has fewer lumina. Sperms are*

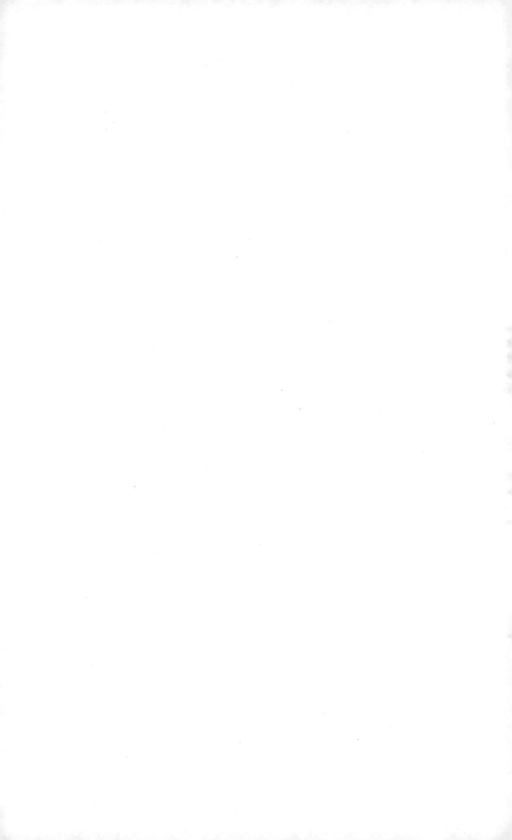

rare or absent in the secretion of the seminal vesicles but are common in the secretion of the ampulla.

F. Ejaculatory Ducts of Ductus Deferens

1. Epithelium is simple columnar or pseudostratified.
2. Mucous membrane forms many thin folds reaching far into the lumen; its connective tissue is provided with abundant elastic networks.
3. The ducts are surrounded by connective tissue.

G. Seminal Vesicles

1. Epithelium shows variations which probably depend on age and functional influences. *It is usually pseudostratified but may be columnar, varying from one to two layers.*
2. *Mucous membrane, much folded, with the folds uniting to form a reticulated surface.*
3. *Vesicles may contain a granular secretion which stains strongly with eosin.*
4. Muscular walls consist chiefly of circular muscles, external to which there may be scattered longitudinal fibers.
5. Sections of the seminal vesicles can be distinguished from gallbladder by the fact that they have a thinner muscular coat than that of gallbladder.

H. Prostate Gland

1. *Epithelium in most places is simple columnar or pseudostratified. In large alveolar cavities it may be low cuboidal or even squamous.*
2. *Mucous membrane much corrugated in appearance.*
3. Alveoli may contain a finely granular secretion.
4. Lamellated, concentric, pink concretions (corpora amylacea) frequently found in the alveoli. Lamellations not always evident. More numerous after middle age.
5. *Fibromuscular stroma.* Muscles and connective tissue constitute about one-third or more of organ. *Note particularly the abundance of discrete single muscle fibers arranged in small interlacing bundles.* This is said to be the only region in the body where this feature is found.

I. Bulbourethral (Cowper's) Glands

1. The epithelium is subject to great functional variations. In the enlarged alveoli the cells are usually flat; in the other glandular spaces they vary from cuboidal to columnar.

2. The interstitial connective tissue contains both smooth and striated muscle with elastic nets.

J. Penis

1. The penis proper consists of three cylindrical bodies.
    a. *Two corpora cavernosa penis located dorsally.* The dorsal artery and vein are located in the subcutaneous connective tissue dorsal to the corpora cavernosa penis.
    b. One corpus cavernosum urethrae (corpus spongiosum) ventral in position. Surrounds the urethra.
    c. The tunica albuginea, a fibrous membrane, surrounds each of the cavernous bodies.
2. *Main substance of the organ is erectile tissue,* which consists of large, irregular, endothelium-lined, venous spaces known as cavernous spaces or lacunae. These are surrounded by connective tissue.
3. Glans penis.
    a. The rounded end of the penis is called the glans penis.
    b. It is covered with a stratified squamous epithelium continuous with the lining of the urethra and also peripherally with the skin of the prepuce.
    c. It consists of dense connective tissue containing nets of anastomosing veins, with circular and longitudinal smooth muscles in their walls.
    d. Richly supplied with sensory nerve endings.
    e. The glans penis is covered by a prepuce (foreskin) which is composed of thin skin with a smooth muscle layer in the hypodermis (subcutaneous layer). *Free from hair follicles.* Modified sebaceous glands (glands of Tyson) may be present. Inner surface adjacent to the glans has the character of a mucous membrane.

TABLE 10. SUMMARY OF THE HISTOLOGY OF THE MALE REPRODUCTIVE SYSTEM

	Organ	Epithelium	Muscle Layers	Connective Tissue
T e s t i s	**Seminiferous Tubules**	Special type composed of sustentacular (Sertoli) cells and spermatogenic cells. From periphery to lumen, the germinal cells are spermatogonia, primary spermatocytes, secondary spermatocytes, and spermatids	None	Basement membrane strengthened by lamellated connective tissue
	Tubuli Recti (Straight Tubules)	Simple epithelium which varies from columnar to cuboidal	None	Surrounded by dense connective tissue of mediastinum
	Rete Testis	Cuboidal or simple squamous	None	Surrounded by dense connective tissue of mediastinum
	Ductuli Efferentes	Tall columnar ciliated cells alternating with cuboidal cells, usually nonciliated	Thin circular layer of smooth muscle	Loose connective tissue in spaces between tubules
D u c t s	**Epididymis**	Pseudostratified stereociliated	Circular layer of smooth muscle	Loose connective tissue in spaces between tubules
	Ductus Deferens (Vas Deferens)	Pseudostratified. Near epididymis; same as ductus epididymis	Inner longitudinal, middle circular, and outer longitudinal layers of smooth muscle	Lamina propria of connective tissue which contains extensive elastic networks. Adventitia of connective tissue
	Ampulla of Ductus Deferens	Cuboidal or columnar	Thinner and less regularly arranged than in other parts of ductus deferens	Lamina propria and adventitia
	Ejaculatory Ducts of Ductus Deferens	Simple columnar or pseudostratified	Muscularis present at beginning	Connective tissue provided with extensive elastic networks

TABLE 10. SUMMARY OF THE HISTOLOGY OF THE MALE
REPRODUCTIVE SYSTEM (Continued)

Organ	Epithelium	Muscle Layers	Connective Tissue
Seminal Vesicles	Individual varia-tions. Usually pseudostratified but may be co-lumnar	Smooth muscle fibers, chiefly cir-cular; external to this layer, longi-tudinal fibers may be present	Lamina propria rich in elastic fibers. Wall of ex-ternal connective tissue with elastic nets
Prostate Gland	Shows great varia-tion but usually simple columnar or pseudostrati-fied	Smooth muscle fibers in intersti-tial tissue	Vascular connec-tive tissue with dense elastic net-works beneath epithelium. In-terstitial connec-tive tissue dense with collagenous fibers and elastic networks
Bulbourethral Glands (Cowper's Glands)	Subject to func-tional variations. In enlarged alveoli, usually flattened. In other glandular spaces the cells vary from cuboi-dal to columnar	Striated and smooth muscle in interstitial tissue	Fibroelastic stroma between tubules
Corpora Cavernosa	Blood spaces lined with endothelium	Strands of smooth muscle in parti-tions between cavernous spaces	Collagenous and elastic fibers in tunica albuginea
Corpus Cavernosum Urethrae (Corpus Spongiosum)	Blood spaces lined with endothelium	Smooth muscle fibers in inner layer of albu-ginea. Smooth muscle in septa	Abundant elastic networks in albu-ginea. Numerous elastic fibers in septa
Glans Penis	Stratified squa-mous	Circular and longi-tudinal smooth muscle in walls of veins	Dense connective tissue containing network of anas-tomosing veins

The first four organ rows (Seminal Vesicles, Prostate Gland, Bulbourethral Glands) are grouped under the vertical label **Accessory Glands**; the last three (Corpora Cavernosa, Corpus Cavernosum Urethrae, Glans Penis) under the vertical label **Penis**.

Chapter 18   FEMALE REPRODUCTIVE SYSTEM

A. Ovary

1. CORTEX

a. Germinal epithelium on the surface of the ovary of the embryo is simple cuboidal or columnar, but becomes flattened later in life.

b. *May show follicles containing ova in the following stages of development:*

(1) *Ovum* enclosed by a *primary follicle* consisting of a single layer of flattened or cuboidal follicular cells and surrounded by interstitial tissue.

(2) Follicle showing the beginning of the zone of growth, that is, a large ovum (oocyte) enclosed by a *zona pellucida* which is surrounded by high, cylindrical, radiating, follicular cells. The immediately surrounding stroma is compressed into a *theca folliculi.*

(3) More advanced stage showing further enlarged ovum with a more distinct *zona pellucida* surrounded by a solid mass of columnar, radiating, follicular cells, forming the *corona radiata.* Theca folliculi more developed.

(4) Mature (Graafian) follicle. The follicle becomes greatly enlarged and assumes an ovoid shape. The follicular cells increase, and a follicular cavity (*antrum folliculi*) with its contained fluid (*liquor folliculi*) develops. As this fluid increases, the ovum is pressed to one side, where it is surrounded by an accumulation of follicular cells (*cumulus oophorus*). Elsewhere the follicular cavity has an epithelium of fairly uniform thickness called the *membrana granulosa.* The theca folliculi is divided into the *theca interna* and the *theca externa.*

(5) Summary of the principal structures of a mature Graafian follicle. The layered structures are listed in order from without, inward:

(a) Theca folliculi $\begin{cases} \text{theca externa.} \\ \text{theca interna.} \end{cases}$

(b) Glassy membrane (basement membrane).

(c) Membrana granulosa.

(d) Liquor folliculi filling the antrum folliculi.

(e) Cumulus oophorus (discus proligerus).

(f) Corona radiata.

(g) Zona pellucida (oolemma).

(h) Vitelline membrane.

(i) Egg cytoplasm (vitellus).

(j) Nucleus.

(k) Nucleolus (germinal spot).

c. May show *corpus haemorrhagicum, corpus luteum, or corpus albicans.*

d. *Stroma of the ovarian cortex is a dense connective tissue, which may be arranged in a whorl-like pattern.*

2. MEDULLA

a. *Consists of loose connective tissue* and some smooth muscle cells.

b. *Many thin-walled blood vessels* in the medulla make it highly vascular, in sharp contrast with the cortex.

B. Corpus Luteum of Ovary

The ruptured follicle does not degenerate immediately after ovulation, but is transformed into a yellow glandular structure known as the corpus luteum.

1. The corpus luteum is large enough to be seen without magnification.

2. The lutein cells are polyhedral in form but often without definite cell walls. They are large cells arranged in irregular masses.

3. In the human, large folds surround a central cavity which is filled with loose connective tissue.

C. Oviduct (Uterine or Fallopian Tube)

1. The wall of the oviduct thickens progressively toward the uterus, while the lumen diminishes considerably in this direction (about 8 to 1 mm).

2. The oviduct is four to five inches long and may be divided into four regions:

a. INFUNDIBULUM.

(1) *The mucous membrane is thrown into complicated folds; the folds are fringed (fimbriae).*

b. AMPULLA. Composes about two-thirds of the duct.

(1) *Epithelium is simple columnar, some cells of which are ciliated.*

(2) *Folds are less complex in ampulla than in fimbriated end, hence the lumen is more evident in the ampulla.*

(3) Muscularis consists of inner circular or spiral and outer longitudinal layers of smooth muscle. Muscle coat thinner and more loosely arranged than that of the isthmus.

  c. ISTHMUS. Includes proximal one-third of the duct.

(1) *Folded lumen lined with simple columnar epithelium, some cells of which are ciliated.* Ciliated cells become less numerous near the uterus.

(2) Muscularis consists of an inner circular or spiral and an outer longitudinal layer of smooth muscle. *Circular or spiral layer is best developed.*

(3) Blood vessels are conspicuous in the outer layer of muscle and in the connective tissue.

(4) May show a serous layer with flattened mesothelial cells.

(5) Though the isthmus is about the same size as the ductus deferens and the ureter, it can be distinguished from them as follows: the oviduct alone lacks an inner longitudinal layer of muscle, *the muscularis of the uterine tube is looser than in the ductus deferens,* and the outer longitudinal muscle of the oviduct spreads out into surrounding tissue in a way that is peculiar to it.

  d. INTRAMURAL PORTION

(1) This is a continuation of the canal through the uterine wall.

D. Uterus

1. ENDOMETRIUM (MUCOSA)

  a. BODY (CORPUS) AND FUNDUS during the follicular phase.

(1) *Simple columnar epithelium, may be shorter or taller in places; some cells ciliated; mucous cells absent.*

(2) *Uterine glands are usually straight slender structures.*

(3) Lamina propria around glands contains many nuclei and lymphocytes.

(4) The endometrium of the body and fundus undergoes cyclic changes during the childbearing period. In general these changes are in the nature of preparation for pregnancy. Four phases of activity can be recognized in this endometrial (menstrual) cycle as follows:

(a) Follicular (proliferative, reparative, estrogenic) phase. Period of repair and growth. Endometrium increases from 0.5 to 2 or 3 mm in thickness. Glands become coiled, more numerous, and lengthen.

    (b) Progravid (luteal) phase.

        (1) Uterine glands increase in extent. Blood vessels become engorged and the endometrium is thick and spongy. The glands under the influence of progesterone are actively secreting.

    (c) Ischemic (premenstrual) phase.

        (1) In the nonpregnant cycle, extensive vascular changes occur 13 to 14 days after ovulation. Stroma becomes denser. Closely packed stroma cells, irregularly collapsed glands, and greatly coiled arteries are characteristic of this phase.

    (d) Menstrual phase.

        (1) Sloughing off of the upper three-fourths of the endometrium. Extravasation of blood occurs.

  b. CERVIX

    (1) Mucosa somewhat thicker than that of body and fundus.

    (2) Simple columnar epithelium, ciliated in places. *Glands are of the mucous type,* considerably branched, and may be cystic.

    (3) Epithelium toward vagina is stratified squamous.

    (4) *Lining of tall featherlike folds, plicae palmatae.*

2. MYOMETRIUM (MUSCULARIS)

  a. BODY AND FUNDUS

    (1) *Dense smooth muscle, difficult to distinguish into layers.*

  b. CERVIX

    (1) The cervix is composed mainly of dense fibrous tissue and smooth muscle fibers. On the average, smooth muscle composes only about 15% of its substance.

3. PERIMETRIUM (SEROSA)

  a. Consists of loose fibroelastic connective tissue lined externally by mesothelium.

E. Placenta

1. *The chorionic villi in cross section appear as various sized islands of connective tissue surrounded by a single layer of deeply staining syncytial cells.* In the young human placenta, up to about two and one-half months of gestation, there are two layers of epithelium covering the chorionic villi: an outer syncytial layer and an inner cubical (Langhans') layer.
2. Blood is found inside and outside of the transversely sectioned villi.
3. *The larger villi show a considerable amount of dense connective tissue.*
4. Decidual cells, large nucleated cells with granular contents arising

from the connective tissue of the uterine mucosa, are quite diagnostic.

F. Vagina

1. Serves as a copulatory receptacle and birth canal.
2. Epithelium contains differing amounts of glycogen depending on the periodic increase of estrogen prior to ovulation; fermentation to lactic acid in vaginal fluid is greatest then. Keratohyaline granules appear in the more superficial layers in about the middle of the cycle. The superficial cells which are cast off are faintly acidophilic and have small dark nuclei. The estrous cycle may be determined by vaginal smears. These smears will show the presence or absence of estrogen production.
   a. MUCOSA
      (1) *Unusually thick stratified squamous epithelium with low broad papillae.* Epithelial cells contain clear areas due to unstained glycogen.
      (2) *Mucosa thrown into coarse folds or rugae.*
      (3) No gland present except in unusual instances where a few glands of the cervical type may be found in the posterior part (fornix).
      (4) Lamina propria of dense connective tissue, often containing numerous lymphocytes.
   b. SUBMUCOSA
      (1) Looser connective tissue than lamina propria, and also more vascular.
      (2) Some histologists do not distinguish between a lamina propria and a submucosa in the vagina.
   c. MUSCULARIS
      (1) *Inner circular and outer longitudinal layers of smooth muscle.* Muscle bundles so irregularly arranged that definite layers may not be apparent.
      (2) Vascular spaces between the muscle bundles may give the appearance of erectile tissue.
   d. ADVENTITIA (FIBROSA)
      a. Connective tissue layer on the outside by which the vagina is attached to adjacent structures.

G. Mammary Gland

1. RESTING GLAND
   a. Bulk of gland consists of *dense connective tissue,* with a few scattered groups of ducts and their branches. The dense interlobular stroma is rich in collagenous bundles and fat cells.

Intralobular stroma is composed of loose connective tissue; fat cells absent. The question of whether alveoli are present is unsettled. *The connective tissue is similar to that of the dermis, but it is free from sweat glands and hair follicles.*

b. *Deep-staining islands of ducts in the nonfunctional gland are very characteristic.*

c. Myoepithelial cells between the epithelium and basement membrane are especially prominent near the excretory ducts.

2. **ACTIVE GLAND (DURING LACTATION)**

a. *The active gland shows the alveoli greatly expanded and filled with secretory material. The secretion is eosinophilic.* Connective tissue is rather dense and considerably reduced when the gland becomes active.

b. *Drops of fat in the lumen of alveoli and ducts.*

c. Active mammary gland resembles thyroid, but the presence of ducts distinguishes it from the endocrine gland.

3. **RETROGRESSIVE GLAND**

a. At the end of a period of lactation, a series of retrogressive changes takes place. Glandular structures are greatly reduced or disappear. Connective tissue elements increase, but the gland as a whole does not quite return to its original state because many of the alveoli which formed during pregnancy do not disappear entirely.

4. **INVOLUTION OF GLAND**

a. After menopause glandular elements are further reduced, until in advanced age there are only a few scattered ducts. The connective tissue is decreased by retrogression, and the whole gland becomes much reduced and shrunken.

5. **NIPPLE AND AREOLA**

a. Skin of the nipple and areola has tall complex dermal papillae extending into the epidermis.

b. Epidermis is deeply pigmented, especially after first pregnancy.

c. Smooth muscles are located circularly around both the papilla mammae and along the length of the lactiferous ducts.

d. Areolar glands of Montgomery in papillary area. These are accessory mammary glands; they are modified sweat glands.

e. Along margin of areola are large sweat and sebaceous glands which lack hairs.

TABLE 11. SUMMARY OF THE HISTOLOGY OF THE FEMALE
REPRODUCTIVE SYSTEM

	Organ	Epithelium	Muscle Layers	Connective Tissue
	Ovary	Germinal epithelium	Strands of smooth muscle cells in medulla	Fibroelastic. May be arranged in whorls in cortex. Loose in medulla
	Oviduct (Uterine or Fallopian Tube)	Simple columnar. Some cells are ciliated	Inner circular or spiral and outer longitudinal layers of smooth muscle	Lamina propria consists of loose variety
U t e r u s	Body and Fundus	Simple columnar. Some cells are ciliated	Smooth muscle difficult to distinguish into layers	Fibrous
	Cervix	Simple columnar. Some cells are ciliated. Lower end lined with stratified squamous	Smooth muscle fibers interspersed with fibrous connective tissue	Fibrous
	Vagina	Stratified squamous	Inner circular and outer longitudinal layers of smooth muscle. Striated muscle fibers form sphincter near orifice	Fibrous

Chapter 19   ENDOCRINE SYSTEM

A. Hypophysis (Pituitary Gland)

1. Examined by low power, *the hypophysis is a thickly capsulated gland and can be divided into four parts; three divisions are distinguishable by their general color reaction with eosin and hematoxylin.*
   a. *The pars distalis (anterior lobe) distinctly eosinophilic (pink).*
   b. *The pars intermedia and pars tuberalis tend to be basophilic (blue).*
   c. *The pars nervosa (posterior lobe) staining but little and appearing fibrous rather than cellular.* In early embryonic stages the pars nervosa contains a cavity. In man and many other mammals, the cavity becomes obliterated although it persists in the adult cat.
2. With special staining techniques, the following histologic details of the four parts may be identified:
   a. PARS DISTALIS (ANTERIOR)
      (1) *Chromophil Cells.* These cells as the name implies have an affinity for stain, and are further classified into two types, based on the staining properties of their specific granules.
         (a) *Alpha cells (acidophils, A cells).* The spherical cytoplasmic granules have some affinity for eosin; therefore, most of the cells in routine preparations are acidophilic.
         (b) *Beta cells (basophils, B cells). The cytoplasm of the beta cells, although it may be colored purple red (instead of blue), is generally of a much darker color than that of the alpha cells.* The beta granules are less numerous than the alpha granules in comparable cells.
             It is of help in identifying these two types of cells to know that *beta cells tend to be more numerous toward the periphery of the gland.* Therefore, since they are fewer than alpha cells, they may not be very numerous in the central part of the gland.
      (2) *Chromophobe Cells* (Chief, Principal, Reserve, C Cells).

Some chromophobes may reach the size of chromophil cells, but *typical chromophobes are much smaller than typical chromophils;* hence, in *a group of chromophobes the nuclei are much closer together than they are in an area of chromophils.* The cell borders of the chromophobes are not so distinct as those of the chromophils. *Cytoplasm is usually agranular and pale-staining.*

b. PARS TUBERALIS

(1) This lobe caps the pars distalis. The outstanding structural character is the *longitudinal arrangement of cords and balls of cells which interdigitate with the longitudinally oriented blood vessels. The cells may be arranged to form a follicular-like structure.* The lumens of these contain a "colloid" material similar in appearance and staining reaction to that found in the thyroid follicles.

(2) The main cell component of the pars tuberalis is roughly cuboidal in shape and is faintly basophilic.

c. PARS INTERMEDIA

(1) Rudimentary in man and ape, but in most mammals it appears as a well-developed layer.

(2) Gland consists chiefly of a few rows of moderately sized cells with strongly basophilic granular cytoplasm. (Granules disappear quickly unless fixation is prompt.) Another type of cell, that is pale-staining, may form follicles containing a colloidal substance resembling in appearance the colloid of the thyroid.

(3) Note the narrow space or cleft (interglandular) between the anterior and posterior lobes. With advancing age this tends to be obliterated.

d. PARS NERVOSA (POSTERIOR LOBE)

(1) Structure not well understood in most species; opossum is probably an exception to the general statement.

(2) Besides nerve fibers, the pars nervosa has a mildly cellular appearance in sections stained by ordinary methods. *However, superficially it resembles a section of nervous tissue.*

(3) The cells peculiar to the human pars nervosa are called *pituicytes.* These cells as well as others such as glial and ependymal are indistinct in routine preparations.

(4) There is a large amount of intercellular substance.

B. Thyroid

1. An external layer of fibroelastic connective tissue envelops the gland, constituting a capsule. Connective tissue septa extend into the substance of the gland.

2. *The parenchyma consists of cords, or clumps of cells, and rounded spaces, or follicles (vesicles), bounded by a simple epithelium, usually of cuboidal cells.* Cells of epithelium may vary from nearly flat to high columnar, depending on the activity of the gland. *The nucleus is spherical. Within many follicles there is a hyaline material which stains deeply with eosin, and is termed colloid.*

3. Some epithelial cells are present outside the follicular wall. It is likely they secrete thyrocalcitonin which is antagonistic in action to parahormone.

4. Basement membrane in older animals; and while present in younger animals, it is too thin to be seen with the light microscope. Cells rest on reticular tissue in young animals.

5. *Superficially, the thyroid may resemble certain phases of the mammary gland, but note the absence of ducts in the thyroid. The size of the follicular units may suggest lung but in the thyroid each space is completely closed and thus there are no incomplete septa as in lung.*

6. Some variations occur in the histologic structure of the human thyroid throughout life until advanced age.

C. Parathyroid

1. Separated from the thyroid by a connective tissue capsule.

2. The parenchyma consists of a *mass of densely packed groups of cells which may form a continuous mass of cells or may be arranged in cords,* rarely in follicles. Between cells there is a framework of reticular fibers, with many anastomosing sinusoidal capillaries. Three main types of epithelial cells compose the cords.

   a. *Principal (chief) cells, nongranular, faintly staining, with large vesicular nuclei.*

   b. *Oxyphil (acidophil) cells, with small deep-staining nuclei and eosinophilic cytoplasm. In contrast to principal cells, the cytoplasm is granular.* Somewhat larger and not nearly so numerous as principal cells.

   c. "Water clear" cells, large cells with cytoplasm that does not take a stain.

3. Isolated or islands of fat cells frequently present in glands of older people.

4. *Superficially may resemble lymphatic tissue, but cells in parathyroid are larger and have more cytoplasm.* Furthermore, they can be recognized as definitely epithelial in nature when examined under high power.

5. Occasionally embedded in the thyroid gland.

6. Gland varies in histologic structure with age.

D. Adrenal (Suprarenal) Glands

1. A connective tissue capsule surrounds the gland.
2. *The gland is distinctly divided into cortex and medulla.*
3. The *cortex* is divided into the following zones:
    a. ZONA GLOMERULOSA. An outer zone lying immediately beneath the capsule. *Consists of short columnar cells in closely packed ovoid groups or in columns.*
    b. ZONA FASCICULATA. *A middle zone in which the cells are arranged in fairly straight cords which run at right angles to the surface.* Cytoplasm of the polyhedral cells may appear *vacuolated* due to lipid droplets having been dissolved.
    c. ZONA RETICULARIS. An inner zone which abuts on the medulla, and in which the cells are in the form of *branching and anastomosing cords.*
4. *The medulla is the more loosely arranged central portion of the gland which stains darker with hematoxylin than the cortex. It consists of irregular cells arranged in rounded groups or short cords* surrounded by venules and blood capillaries.
    a. The cytoplasm contains a number of specific secretory granules, which are precursors of the hormone epinephrine. These granules turn brown by contact with an appropriate oxidizing agent; the effect is known as the chromaffin reaction.
    b. The vascular supply is richest of any organ in the body.
    c. Unmyelinated nerves enter capsule in small bundles; some end in the cortex but most end about medullary cells.

E. Islets of Langerhans (Pancreatic Islands)

1. Spheroidal aggregations of pale-staining polyhedral cells.
2. With special fixation and staining, three distinct types of cells have been demonstrated: (1) alpha cells, fairly numerous in most islands; granules soluble in water; (2) beta cells, smaller and still more numerous, alcohol soluble; and (3) delta cells, the rarest. There is a question as to whether delta cells are a separate cell or part of a developmental stage.
3. *Not acinous in character like the rest of the pancreas.*

F. Corpus Luteum of Ovary

1. Described on p. 182.

G. Interstitial Cells of Testis

1. Described on p. 170.

H. Pineal Body (Epiphysis)

1. Fibrous capsule formed by the pia mater.
2. *Numerous fibrous tissue processes and septa pass into the gland from the capsule which more or less divide the gland into lobules.*
3. The pineal cells are mainly apparent by their nuclei when stained with H. and E. Five types of cells have been described when special staining methods were used.
4. *"Brain-sand granules" (corpora arenacea; psammoma bodies), dark laminated, calcareous concretions, may be conspicuous.* These calcareous bodies may not be present in earliest infancy.

I. Thymus

1. This organ is sometimes discussed with the endocrine glands. There is some evidence that it produces a humoral factor which stimulates the production of lymphocytes, and perhaps the immunologic competence of lymphocytes. The evidence, however, is only suggestive.

Chapter 20   EYE

A. Cornea

It is composed of five layers which from without inward are:

1. **CORNEAL EPITHELIUM.** On the anterior surface it is stratified squamous.
2. **BOWMAN'S MEMBRANE (ANTERIOR ELASTIC MEMBRANE).** This is a fibrillated membrane on which the corneal epithelium rests. This membrane does not contain elastin.
3. **SUBSTANTIA PROPRIA (CORNEAL STROMA).** This forms about 90% of the thickness of the cornea. Consists mostly of collagenous fibers which are arranged in lamellae running parallel to the surface.
4. **DESCEMET'S MEMBRANE (POSTERIOR ELASTIC MEMBRANE).** It is a basement membrane on the anterior surface of the corneal mesenchymal epithelium.
5. **CORNEAL MESENCHYMAL EPITHELIUM (CORNEAL ENDOTHELIUM).** This is composed of thick squamous cells. The cornea proper is devoid of blood vessels, which may be the reason it can be transplanted from one individual to another.

B. Sclera (Tunica Fibrosa)

1. **EPISCLERAL TISSUE**
   a. The outermost layer composed of loose collagenous and elastic fibers. It differs from the sclera proper in having a relatively large number of blood vessels.
2. **EXTERNAL LAYER (SCLERA PROPER)**
   a. This layer consists of elastic and flat collagenous fibers which run in various directions parallel to the surface.
3. **INTERNAL LAYER (LAMINA FUSCA)**
   a. Contains a varying number of branched pigment cells. More elastic fibers than in the external layer.

C. Choroid

From without inward the following layers can be distinguished.

1. **SUPRACHOROID LAYER (LAMINA SUPRACHORIOIDEA)**
   a. Thin membranes (lamellae) of fine connective tissue containing chromatophores between and in the membranes.
2. **VESSEL LAYER (LAMINA VASCULOSA)**
   a. Consists of numerous large and medium-sized arteries and veins. The spaces between vessels are filled with *loose connective tissue* rich in chromatophores.
3. **CAPILLARY LAYER (CHORIOCAPILLARIS LAYER)**
   a. Consists of a capillary network.
4. **BRUCH'S (GLASSY) MEMBRANE (LAMINA VITREA)**
   Under most favorable conditions two layers may be distinguished:
   a. OUTER LAYER
      (1) Thin layer of elastic fibers.
   b. INNER LAYER
      (1) Homogeneous and thicker than outer.

D. Ciliary Body

Six layers may be described in the ciliary body. From without inward they are:

1. **SUPRACHOROID AND CILIARY MUSCLE.** The suprachoroid and ciliary muscle make up the bulk of the ciliary body. The muscle fibers are oriented in three directions: meridional, radial, and circular layers.
2. **VESSEL LAYER.** It consists for the most part of veins.
3. **GLASSY MEMBRANE (LAMINA VITREA).** Continuous with the same structure in the choroid but consists of three layers.
4. **PIGMENT EPITHELIUM.** It is a continuation of the pigment layer of the retina.
5. **CILIARY EPITHELIUM.** It represents a continuation of the sensory portion of the retina.
6. **INTERNAL LIMITING MEMBRANE.** This is a very thin structureless membrane.

E. Iris

1. **ANTERIOR SURFACE OF STROMA**
   a. Covered by a single layer of mesenchymal epithelium and sometimes termed the *endothelium* of the iris. Difficult to demonstrate in sections.

2. ANTERIOR STROMAL SHEET (OR LAMELLA)

a. Consists of a homogeneous ground substance, few collagenous fibers, and many fibroblasts and chromatophores. The amount of pigment varies from none to large amounts.

3. VESSEL LAYER

a. Contains many blood vessels between which are loose connective tissue and some branched chromatophores.

4. MUSCLES OF IRIS

a. The iris contains two smooth muscles: (1) circular sphincter of the pupil and (2) the dilator of the pupil. The fibers of these muscles are not typical of smooth muscle and are called by some authors myoepithelial cells.

5. POSTERIOR PART OF IRIS

a. The *pigment epithelium* forming the posterior layer of the iris consists of a layer of columnar epithelial cells. In ordinary preparations the dark brown granules of melanin obscure the cell boundaries.

F. Retina. Largely of nervous elements.

1. VISUAL PORTION (PARS OPTICA). From without inward the following layers can be distinguished:

  a. PIGMENTED EPITHELIAL LAYER
    (1) Consists of hexagonal-shaped cells when seen from the surface which contain the *pigment fuscin.*
  b. LAYER OF RODS AND CONES
    (1) Consists of *elongated, cylindrical-shaped rod cells,* and shorter, thicker *cone cells.*
  c. EXTERNAL (OUTER) LIMITING MEMBRANE
  d. OUTER NUCLEAR (GRANULAR) LAYER
    (1) *Nuclei of the rod and cone cells present.*
  e. OUTER PLEXIFORM (MOLECULAR, RETICULAR) LAYER
    (1) Fibrous.
  f. INNER NUCLEAR (GRANULAR) LAYER
    (1) Cell bodies and *nuclei* of various cells.
  g. INNER PLEXIFORM (MOLECULAR) LAYER
    (1) Fibrous.
  h. LAYER OF GANGLION CELLS
  i. LAYER OF OPTIC NERVE FIBERS
  j. INNER LIMITING MEMBRANE

G. Lens

1. Surface of lens is covered by a homogeneous capsule.
2. Within the capsule the anterior surface of the lens is lined by an

epithelium of a single layer of cuboidal cells which are taller toward the equator where they approach a columnar form.
3. Lens fibers consist of elongated six-sided (hexagonal) prisms.

H. Vitreous Body

1. In fresh condition the substance of the vitreous body has a gelatinous consistency. In fixed sections it shows a network of extremely fine fibrils with its meshes filled with a clear liquid.

I. Optic Nerve

1. CROSS SECTION OF ENTIRE NERVE

   a. *Large bundles of transversely cut nerve fibers, large and myelinated, but without neurolemma.* These fibers pass through the lamina cribrosa before acquiring their myelin sheaths.
   b. *Fibers are grouped into bundles completely separated by connective tissue septa.*
   c. Surrounded from within outward by pia mater, arachnoid, and dura mater membranes.
   d. Subdural space is relatively large.
   e. Middle portion of optic nerve occupied by *central artery* and *central vein.*

J. Eyelids

1. *Tarsal plate* is a layer of very dense connective tissue which supports the lid.
2. *Tarsal (Meibomian) glands. These are complex sebaceous glands. Each consists of a long straight central duct surrounded by numerous alveoli which open into it.*
3. Hair follicles usually present.
4. The *conjunctiva* (mucous membrane) is the innermost layer of the eyelid.

K. Lacrimal Glands

1. This gland bears a very close resemblance to the parotid gland, but differs as follows:
   a. *The lumina of the alveoli are generally larger than in the parotid.*
   b. Dark-staining glandular cells have typically a narrower columnar shape than those of the parotid.
   c. Between the glandular cells and the basement membrane are numerous basket (myoepithelial) cells.

Chapter 21   EAR

A. External Ear

1. AURICLE (PINNA)
a. *Elastic cartilage in center.*
b. *Connective tissue outside the cartilage.*
c. Thin skin on both sides with hair follicles and sebaceous glands.
d. Sweat glands are scarce and small.

2. EXTERNAL AUDITORY MEATUS
a. In its outer part, walls are formed by continuation of the cartilage of the auricle and in the inner portion by the temporal bone.
b. Thin skin lines the walls. Hair follicles, sebaceous glands, and *ceruminous glands* are present in the outer part.

3. TYMPANIC MEMBRANE (EARDRUM)
This is a thin membrane which separates the external ear from the middle ear. Some authors classify it as a part of the middle ear.
a. The outer surface is lined by a thin layer of skin.
b. The fibrous portion between the outer and inner epithelia consists of collagenous fibers and a thin network of elastic fibers. The outer layer is radially arranged. The inner layer is circularly arranged.
c. The inner surface is covered by a single layer of flattened squamous epithelium.

B. Middle Ear

1. TYMPANIC CAVITY
a. The epithelium is generally simple squamous. In several places, especially near the opening of the auditory tube and near the edge of the tympanic membrane, it is cuboidal or columnar.
b. The three ear bones or *auditory ossicles* are in this cavity. From the exterior to interior they are *malleus, incus,* and *stapes.*

2. AUDITORY (EUSTACHIAN) TUBE
a. BONY OR OSSEOUS PART
   (1) Epithelium is low columnar ciliated.

   b. CARTILAGINOUS PART
      (1) In the portion nearer the pharynx, the epithelium is pseu-
           dostratified ciliated.
      (2) At pharyngeal opening numerous goblet cells appear.

C. Inner Ear (Labyrinth)

1. VESTIBULE
   a. This is an irregular, oval-shaped cavity.
   b. The lateral wall, which forms the medial wall of the tympanic
      cavity, is pierced by two small openings, or "windows": the
      fenestra cochlea (round opening) and the fenestra ovalis (oval
      opening).
2. SACCULE
   a. This saclike structure occupies the lower anterior part of the
      vestibule.
   b. The outer layer consists of fine connective tissue, in which
      branched pigment cells are often found.
   c. The epithelium, which is flattened, is separated from the con-
      nective tissue by a distinct membrane.
   d. Maculae present.
3. UTRICLE
   a. This has an oblong, transversely compressed form, and occupies
      the upper posterior part of the vestibule. This is larger than the
      saccule.
   b. Structure same as that of the saccule.
4. SEMICIRCULAR CANALS
   a. These three canals are long loop-shaped tubes. Each lies in a
      different plane; namely, the superior (frontal), the posterior
      (sagittal), and the lateral (horizontal).
   b. Structurally the walls are similar to those of the utricle and
      saccule.
5. AMPULLA
   a. This is the dilated end of a semicircular canal.
   b. In a longitudinal section of the ampulla the crista is cut in
      cross section and appears as a high rounded prominence occupy-
      ing about one third of the lumen.
   c. When cut longitudinally, the *crista* is seen to be highest in its
      middle part, and slopes down toward the side walls of the
      ampulla.
6. BONY COCHLEA
   a. This is a spirally coiled tube which resembles a snail shell.
   b. Connects to the anterior wall of the vestibule.

7. ORGAN OF CORTI

   a. This is the sensory part of the organ of hearing and forms a thick ridge which runs along the cochlear duct.

   b. In radial section it has the form of an irregular trapezoid prominence bulging into the lumina of the cochlear duct.

   c. There are different types of *supporting cells* but all appear *tall and slender,* extending from the basilar membrane to the free surface of the organ of Corti.

   d. The *hair (neuroepithelial) cells* on the free surface have short, rigid, bristlelike outgrowths. The two types of hair cells, *inner* and *outer,* are short cylinders with rounded lower ends that contain a nucleus.

8. TECTORIAL MEMBRANE

   a. The surface of the organ of Corti is covered by a ribbonlike gelatinous structure, called the *tectorial membrane.*

   b. Composed of a homogeneous ground substance with numerous fibrils.

Chapter 22   OLFACTORY ORGAN

A. Olfactory Epithelium

1. EPITHELIUM

It is of the pseudostratified columnar type. The surface cells are of three kinds.

a. SUPPORTING CELLS (SUSTENTACULAR)

(1) These are tall slender cells.

(2) *The nuclei are oval in shape. Two or three rows of these oval nuclei are seen in sections.*

b. BASAL CELLS

(1) These cells lie between the bases of the supporting cells.

(2) Basal cells are more or less triangular, with dark nuclei and branching processes.

c. OLFACTORY CELLS

(1) Bipolar nerve cells of fusiform shape with *several rows of spherical nuclei.*

(2) The round nuclei occupy a zone between the nuclei of the supporting cells and the nuclei of the basal cells.

(3) A cylindrical process, a modified dendrite, extends from the peripheral part of each cell to the surface. At the surface, each dendrite becomes expanded to form an *olfactory vesicle;* and from this, delicate processes called *olfactory hairs* extend from the surface.

(4) Basally the olfactory cell tapers into a filament, actually an axon.

2. LAMINA PROPRIA

a. Connective tissue consists of collagenous and elastic fibers. Contains a rich plexus of blood capillaries. In the deep layers there is a *plexus of large veins* and lymph capillaries.

b. *Bowman's glands* (olfactory).

(1) These are in the lamina propria.

(2) They are of the tubuloalveolar type and the cuboidal glandular cells *resemble serous cells.*

Chapter 23   TASTE (GUSTATORY) ORGAN

The organ of taste consists of the taste buds of the mucosa of the tongue; a few may be present in other parts of the mouth and in the lining of the throat.

A. Structure of Taste Buds

1. These are little barrel-shaped groups of cells embedded in the stratified epithelium in which they occur. Each taste bud is connected with the surface by a small opening, the *gustatory pore.* Two types of epithelium are present:

   a. SUPPORTING (SUSTENTACULAR) CELLS

   (1) These are spindle-shaped, and their ends surround a small opening, the *inner taste pore,* which leads into a pitlike excavation. They are roughly parallel to the bud axis, that is, they are arranged like the sections of an orange.

   b. TASTE (NEUROEPITHELIAL, GUSTATORY) CELLS

   (1) Long spindle-shaped cells ending in hairlike processes which project freely into the lumen of the pit. The *elongated dark-staining nuclei are placed in the midportions of the cells.* These cells are centrally located and parallel to the long axis of the bud.

Chapter 24   TISSUES AND ORGANS SOMETIMES CONFUSED

The tissues and organs listed after each number below are those which beginning students of histology may mistake one for the other. This list has been prepared from incorrect answers given by students on final histologic laboratory tests in identification. Special study of this list should greatly lessen errors in the microscopic identification of tissues and organs.

1. Thymus, lymph gland, hemolymph gland, spleen, parathyroid.
2. Lung, bone marrow, mucous tissue, mammary gland, thyroid.
3. Cartilage, cerebral cortex.
4. Vagina, esophagus, bladder, pharynx, oviduct.
5. Oviduct (isthmus), ductus efferens, ureter, urethra.
6. Oviduct (ampulla), seminal vesicle, gallbladder.
7. Ductulus efferens, epididymis.
8. Ligamentum nuchae, heart muscle, pregnant uterus.
9. Corpus luteum, adrenal.
10. Smooth muscle, nerve, fibrous connective tissue, elastic tissue.
11. Prostate, seminal vesicle, gallbladder, fimbriated extremity of oviduct.
12. Parotid gland, pancreatic gland, sublingual gland, submaxillary gland, lacrimal gland.
13. Aorta, ligamentum nuchae, nerve.
14. Pharynx, tongue, bladder, uterus.
15. Mammary gland, thyroid gland, lacrimal gland, Cowper's gland, prostate gland.
16. Lymph gland, tonsil, thymus, spleen.
17. Heart muscle, skeletal muscle, smooth muscle.
18. Vein, artery, lymph vessel.
19. Corpus luteum, decidua vera (parietalis).
20. Stomach, small intestine, large intestine.
21. Lip, lower cutaneous border of anus.
22. Stretched transitional epithelium, stratified squamous epithelium.
23. Stratified columnar epithelium, pseudostratified epithelium.
24. Bronchioles, arteries.

25. Esophagus stomach junction, anorectal junction, vertical section of lip.
26. Myelinated nerve, unmyelinated nerve fibers.
27. Mucous tissue, mesenchyme.
28. Oviduct, small intestine, appendix.
29. Skin, vagina, esophagus.
30. White fibrocartilage, elastic cartilage.

Chapter 25   SUMMARY OF MAIN DISTRIBUTION OF CARTILAGE

A. Hyaline Cartilage

1. Preforms all bones except flat bones of face and skull.
2. Nasal cartilages.
3. Most of the laryngeal cartilages.
4. Tracheal and bronchial cartilages.
5. Costal cartilages.
6. Some articular cartilages.
7. Epiphyseal cartilages until epiphysis joins diaphysis and xiphoid process.

B. Yellow Elastic Cartilage

1. Auricle (pinna).
2. Eustachian tube.
3. Epiglottis.
4. Part of arytenoid, corniculate, and cuneiform cartilages.

C. White Fibrocartilage

1. Intervertebral disks.
2. Some articular cartilages.
3. Symphysis pubis.
4. Ligamentum teres of femur.
5. Glenoid ligament of shoulder and cotyloid ligament of hip.
6. Interarticular cartilages of many joints as the clavicle, sternum, lower jaw, knee, etc.
7. Lines tendon grooves of the bones.
8. Junction of tendon and bone.

GLOSSARY

ac′id dye   A salt of a mineral base (generally sodium) and an organic acid that is colored. In solution it is negatively charged.

a·cid′o·phil″   A cell having an affinity for acid stains. Includes alpha cells found in the anterior pituitary body and those in the adenohypophysis.

ac′i·nus   A sacular terminal division of a compound gland having a narrow lumen. Often used synonymously with alveolus.

ad″a·man′to·blast   An enamel-forming cell. Synonyms: ameloblast, ganoblast.

ad″e·no·hy·poph′y·sis   The glandular part of the pituitary gland developing from somatic ectoderm of the posterior nasopharynx.

ad″ven·ti′ti·a   The external covering of an organ derived from adjacent connective tissue.

af′fer·ent   Carrying toward.

al·ve′o·lus   The terminal portion of a gland that is spherical or oval and possesses a conspicuous lumen. An air cell of the lung. Sometimes used synonymously with acinus.

a·mel′o·blast   An enamel-forming cell. Synonyms: adamantoblast, ganoblast.

am·pul′la of Vater   The dilatation of the common bile duct and pancreatic duct where they join the duodenum.

a·nas′to·mose   To join by connecting branches, as nerves, or to open one into another, as blood vessels and lymphatics.

ap′a·tite   A type of mineral, a form of which is found in the inorganic compound of bones and teeth.

ap′o·crine gland   A gland that produces its secretion by disintegration of the free ends of the cells.

a·re′o·la   1. Any minute interstice or space in a tissue. 2. A colored or pigmented ring surrounding some central point or space as a nipple. 3. The part of the iris enclosing the eye.

a·re′o·lar tis′sue   A connective tissue composed of white and yellow elastic fibers that interlace in all directions, forming a loose meshwork.

ar·gen′taf·fin   Referring to the capacity of certain tissue elements to reduce silver in staining solution.

ar·gen′taf·fin cells   Cells in all parts of the alimentary tract from the esophagus to the anus, but most numerous in the small intestine. Their cytoplasm contains argyrophilic granules. These cells are located between the cells lining the glands of Lieberkühn.

ar·gy″ro·phil′ic   Having an affinity for silver.

ar′te·fact, ar′ti·fact   In histology and microscopy, tissue that has been mechanically altered from its natural state; also, anything that has not been present normally.

a·ryt′e·noid   Resembling the mouth of a pitcher. Pertaining to the arytenoid cartilage, glands, and muscles.

as′tro·cytes   The many-processed stellate cells of the neuroglia attached to the blood vessels of the brain and spinal cord by perivascular feet.

at′ro·phy   Diminution in size of a cell, tissue, organ, or part thereof.

Auer′bach's plex′us   Myenteric plexus and the ganglion cells found therein.

au·tol′y·sis   The self-digestion of cells by the action of their own enzymes.

a·zu″ro·phil′ic   Having an affinity for an azure dye.

base′ment mem′brane   The delicate noncellular membrane on which an epithelium is seated; also called basal membrane, membrana propria.

ba′sic dye   A mineral salt (generally chloride) of a colored organic base. In solution it bears a positive charge.

ba′so·phil   A substance, cell, or tissue element showing an affinity for basic dyes. Leukocytes somewhat larger than an erythrocyte. The nucleus is usually bent in the form of an S and is provided with two or more constrictions. The cytoplasm contains very large irregular granules which stain a deep blue-violet color. Also, one of the beta cells found in the adenohypophysis.

Bow′man's cap′sule   The invaginated portion of the beginning of the uriniferous tubule.

brain sand   Psammoma bodies in the pineal body. Corpora arenacea.

Brun′ner's glands   Submucosal glands in the wall of the duodenum in the region of the pyloric sphincter.

brush bor′der   Nonmotile, hairlike outgrowths that stand upright, in the fashion of a dense brush, on the free surface of an epithelium. Electron microscope shows that the appearance of a brush border is due to regular foldings of the plasma membrane.

bul″bo·u·re′thral glands   Pea-sized structures situated on either side of the urethral bulb and connected with the urethra by long ducts. Also called Cowper's glands.

cell   A spatially limited mass of protoplasm, with few exceptions, which contains a nucleus. The cell is the structural, functional, hereditary, and developmental unit of life. It is the minimal structural unit of protoplasm in an organism that can carry on all of the vital functions.

cell mem′brane   The outer limit of a cell consisting of three layers and composed of a lipoprotein complex. Synonyms: plasma membrane, plasmalemma.

cen′tri·ole A minute body, rod, or granule, usually found in the centrosome and frequently considered to be the active, self-perpetuating, division center of the cell.

cen″tro·ac′i·nous cells Cells of the terminals of the intralobular ducts continued into the acini of the pancreas.

cen′tro·some The centrosphere together with the centriole or centrioles.

cen′tro·sphere″ A hyaline body of differentiated cytoplasm found at the center of the astral rays in mitosis and meiosis.

cer″e·bel′lum The inferior part of the brain lying below the cerebrum and above the pons and medulla, consisting of two lateral lobes and a middle lobe.

cer′e·brum The largest portion of the brain occupying the whole upper part of the cranium and consisting of the right and left hemispheres.

chor′da ten′din·ea Any one of the tendons of the papillary muscles of the ventricles of the heart attached to the atrioventricular valves.

chro′ma·tin The substance of the nucleus of a cell that specifically stains by a method called the Feulgen reaction. It contains deoxyribonucleic acid, the genetic material.

chro′mo·phil substance (Nissl bodies) Consists of discrete clumps in living cells that belong to the chromidial group in the system of endoplasmic reticulum. By electron microscopy they consist of ribonucleoprotein (RNP, ribosomes), which is both free and associated with the endoplasmic reticulum.

chro′mo·phobe cell A cell which does not stain easily. Cell of the adenohypophysis.

chro′mo·some Any one of the separate, deeply staining bodies, which are commonly rod-, J-, or V-shaped, which become evident from the nuclear network during mitosis, and which split longitudinally in the course of that process. They carry the heredity factors (genes) and are present in constant numbers in each species.

cil′i·a A motile form of the specialization of the surface of the cell. Usually numerous in number and short in length.

cir″cum·a′nal Surrounding the anus.

clas·mat′o·cyte Macrophage. A phagocytic cell belonging to the reticuloendothelial system.

coc″cy·ge′al body This body is located in front of the apex of the coccyx; it consists of numerous arteriovenous anastomoses with a relatively thick wall embedded in dense fibrous connective tissue.

Cohn′heim′s a′re·as or fields Myofibrils arranged in small groups as seen in cross section. Also called Kölliker′s areas or fields.

col·lag′e·nous (white) fibers Extremely fine, 1 to 12 microns in thickness, white fibers whose course is characteristically wavy. Collagenous fibers are arranged in bundles. By electron microscopy, they are characteristically cross-banded.

col'loid A state of subdivision of matter in which the particles are dispersed in, or distributed throughout, a medium called the dispersion medium, such as a liquid, gas, or solid.

con·nec'tive tis'sue A tissue composed of cells and certain other material produced by the cells, that in its simple form binds organs and tissues together. It is typically relatively rich in extracellular material and poor in cells. In a broader sense, it includes cartilage and bone; blood may also be considered a connective tissue.

cor·nic'u·late In the form of a horn. Horn-shaped appendages.

cor'ni·fied Converted by a process of differentiation into dead, horny, protective layers.

co·ro'na A crown.

co·ro'na ra"di·a'ta A zone of follicular cells circumjacent to the zona pellucida of the ovum, which persists for some time after ovulation.

cor'pus 1. The body. 2. The largest and, primarily, the central part of an organ.

cor'pus lu'te·um The yellow endocrine body formed in the ovary at the site of a ruptured Graafian follicle.

cor'tex The peripheral zone of an organ in contrast with its central zone.

cor'ti·cal Relating to the cortex.

cre'nat·ed Notched or scalloped. Crenated corpuscles are shrunken erythrocytes, on the surface of which are spiny or knoblike processes.

cri'coid The signet-ring-shaped cartilage of the larynx.

cross sec'tion A section cut from a structure across, crosswise, or transverse to the long axis. Synonym: transection.

crypts of Lie'ber·kühn Simple straight tubular glands of the intestinal mucous membrane; slits from the base of the duodenal villi that extend into the mucosa as far as the muscularis mucosae. Excretory ducts of Brunner's gland usually open into these crypts. Also called intestinal glands, mucous crypts.

cu'mu·lus o·oph'o·rus The mass of follicular cells surrounding the ovum and protruding into the liquid-filled cavity of a Graafian follicle.

cu·ne'i·form Wedge-shaped.

cu'ti·cle A horny or chitinous, sometimes calcified, layer formed by and covering an epithelium; it is formed as a secretion of the cytoplasm.

cy"to·gen'e·sis Cell development or reproduction.

cy"to·gen'ic glands Glands that produce a secretion, parts of which are living cells.

cy·tol'o·gy The science that deals with the study of cells.

cy"to·mor'pho·sis The series of changes in a cell from its formation through destruction.

cy'to·plasm The protoplasm of a cell, excluding the nucleus.

dem′i·lune A crescent-shaped aggregation of serous cells capping mucous cells in mixed glands.

de·ox″y·ri″bo·nu′cle·ic ac′id (DNA) Genetic material in chromatin.

des′mo·cyte Any kind of supporting tissue cell.

des′mo·some A thickening in the middle of an intercellular bridge in epidermis.

dip′lo·some The pair of centrioles commonly found in certain cells.

DNA (deoxyribonucleic acid) Genetic material in chromatin.

duc′tu·li ef″fer·en′tes Ductules leading from the rete testis to the epididymis.

duc′tus def′er·ens The portion of the excretory duct system of the testis which runs from the epididymal duct to the ejaculatory duct.

duc′tus ep″i·did′y·mis Epididymal duct.

ef′fer·ent Carrying away.

e·las′tic fi′bers Homogeneous branched fibers that anastomose into loose networks. They are much thinner than collagenous fibers and have a yellowish color in living tissue. They are elastic and are often curled at their free ends.

en·am′el The dense white covering of the crown of a tooth. It is mineralized protein with a prismatic structure. It is the hardest substance in the animal body.

en″do·car′di·um The membrane lining the interior of the heart, consisting of endothelium and the subjacent connective tissue.

en″do·chon′dral Situated within a cartilage.

en″do·neu′ri·um The delicate connective tissue holding together the fibers of a nerve bundle.

en′do·plas″mic re·tic′u·lum Consists of the cytoplasmic membranes continuous with the plasma membranes and the outer nuclear membrane.

en″do·the′li·um The cellular membrane that lines the blood vessels, heart, and lymphatic vessels.

e″o·sin′o·phil Leukocytes about twice the size of an erythrocyte; nucleus often has two oval lobes connected by a nuclear thread. The cytoplasm contains coarse refractive granules which stain a red color.

ep·en′dy·ma The lining membrane of the cerebral ventricles and the central canal of the spiral cord.

ep″i·car′di·um The visceral layer of the pericardium.

ep″i·neu′ri·um The connective tissue sheath of a nerve trunk.

ep″i·phys′e·al car′ti·lage The plate of cartilage between the epiphysis and main portion of the bone.

ep″i·the′li·um Usually a group of cells covering a surface; the cells are close together with little extracellular connective tissue. Those exceptions that appear in the form of solid masses or follicles also have their embryologic origin from a surface tissue.

ep″o·nych′i·um   The horny layer of the nail fold attached to the nail plate at its margin.

er·gas′to·plasm   That part of the endoplasmic reticulum which consists of the networks of canaliculi, flattened sacs and vacuoles that have a limiting membrane, and dense granules of ribonucleoprotein spaced along the outer surfaces of the membrane. It may also include free ribosomes.

e·ryth′ro·cyte   The nonnucleated and agranular cell of human blood whose oxygen-carrying pigment, hemoglobin, is responsible for the red color of fresh blood. Cell is generally disk-shaped and biconcave.

e·ryth″ro·plas′tid   An erythrocyte. The nonnucleated and agranular cell of human blood whose oxygen-carrying pigment, hemoglobin, is responsible for the red color of fresh blood.

ex·trav″a·sa′tion   The passing of a fluid, such as blood, from its proper vessel into surrounding tissue.

fac′et   A small face, usually of some geometrical form.

fas′ci·a   A fibroelastic tissue that surrounds and connects the muscles.

fas·cic′u·lus   A bundle of close-set fibers, usually muscle or nerve fibers.

fe·nes′trat·ed   Having windowlike openings.

fi′ber   A threadlike structure of organic tissue.

fi′bril, fi·bril′la   A minute component filament of a fiber; it is a characteristic structure in nerve and muscle cells.

fi′bro·blast   A common connective tissue cell. It is a flattened, irregularly branched cell with a large oval nucleus. It produces collagen. Synonyms: desmocyte, fibrocyte.

fi″bro·e·las′tic tis′sue   Connective tissue composed of both white (collagenous) and yellow (elastic) fibers.

fla·gel′lum   A whiplike process consisting of an axial filament enclosed in a thin cytoplasmic sheath. Flagella are usually long and few in number as compared to cilia.

fol′li·cle   A small secretory cavity or sac.

fu·nic′u·lus   A small cordlike structure such as one of the bundles of nerve fibers, the aggregate of which composes a nerve trunk.

fu′si·form   Spindle-shaped.

gan′gli·on   A group or mass of nerve-cell bodies (cytons) usually located outside the central nervous system.

gan′o·blast   An enamel-forming cell. Synonyms: adamantoblast, ameloblast.

gen″i·ta′li·a   The genitals (includes the organs of reproduction).

ger′mi·nal cen′ter   A pale-staining area of active mitosis in the center of a lymph nodule or follicle where the lymphocytes are loosely packed. The area is associated with the production of antibodies.

gin'gi·va That part of the oral mucous membrane which surrounds the tooth distal to the alveolar crest.

gland One or many associated cells that secrete or excrete a special substance.

gli'a The neuroglia.

glo·mer'u·lus A small coiled mass of capillaries contained in Bowman's capsule of the kidney.

gob'let cell An epithelial cell that secretes mucus.

Gol'gi ap"pa·ra'tus A network of fibers or canals found in the cytoplasm of cells. These fibers or canals, which may take the form of rods, granules, or spheres, react selectively to osmic acid. In electron micrographs the Golgi apparatus consists of parallel arrays of membranes and small vesicles. It is secretory in function.

Graaf'i·an fol'li·cle The mature ovarian follicle.

gran'u·lo·cyte" A granular leukocyte; a polymorphonuclear leukocyte, either eosinophilic, basophilic, or neutrophilic.

hair fol'li·cle The depression containing the root of a hair.

H. and E. Abbreviation for hematoxylin and eosin stain.

Has'sall's cor'pus·cles Organizations of epithelial cells unique to the thymus.

Ha·ver'si·an ca·nals' The anastomosing canals of the bone, containing blood vessels, lymph vessels, and nerves.

he"ma·tox'y·lin A crystalline compound containing the coloring matter of logwood. It is used as a dye in microtechniques.

het"er·o·ge'ne·ous Not uniform: opposed to homogeneous.

hi'lus A depression at the entrance and exit of vessels, nerves, and ducts into a gland.

his'ti·o·cyte Fixed macrophage of the loose connective tissue. Histiocytes in common with other cells belonging to the reticuloendothelial system, store selectively certain dyes such as trypan blue or lithium carmine. Formerly called resting wandering cell. Sometimes used synonymously with *macrophage*.

his"to·gen'e·sis The origin, development, and differentiation of the tissues of an organism.

his·tol'o·gy That branch of anatomy which deals with the minute structure of tissues and organs and with the morphologic evidence of their functions. General histology is the study of the several fundamental tissues. Special histology deals with the minute structure of the organs.

hol'o·crine gland A gland in which the products accumulate within the cell itself; the cell is discharged as the secretion of the gland.

ho"mo·ge'ne·ous Of uniform structure: opposed to heterogeneous.

hy'a·line Smooth, glassylike in appearance.

hy·per'tro·phy   Excessive growth or development of an organ or part of an organ of an animal.

hy"po·nych'i·um   The thickened stratum corneum of the epidermis which lies under the free edge of a nail.

hy·poph'y·sis   Pituitary gland.

in·ter'ca·la"ted disks   Transverse bands across heart muscle fibers. They may, however, extend only part way across a fiber and may be irregular or broken into step formations. They are usually distinct in H. and E. preparations but can be brought out clearly by staining with silver nitrate or other special stains. By electron microscopy these appear as junctions between cells; they are plasma membrane modified to become much denser than elsewhere. Structurally they are similar to desmosomes.

in·ter'ca·la"ted duct   A very small duct connected with an acinus, or alveolus, of a gland.

in"ter·cel'lu·lar brid'ges   Sites of end-to-end contacts of short processes on adjacent cells. No actual continuity between cells.

in"ter·dig"i·ta'tion   The complex infolding and dovetailing of the plasma membrane, which may be seen in cells closely associated, increasing the surface of plasma membrane, which may facilitate transport of material in or out of cells.

in"ter·lob'u·lar   Situated between lobes.

in"ter·sti'tial   Situated between important parts. Occupying the inter-spaces of a part. Interstitial cells usually occur in dense compact groups of various sizes lying in the stroma of the angular spaces between the tubules.

in"tra·car"ti·lag'i·nous   Within a cartilage.

in"tra·lob'u·lar   Within a lobule.

in"tra·mem'bra·nous   Developing or taking place within a membrane.

je·ju'num   The second division of the small intestine extending between the duodenum and the ileum and measuring about eight feet in length.

ker'a·tin   A horny material, protecting surfaces.

Kupf'fer cells   Fixed macrophages lining the sinusoids of the liver.

la'bi·al   Relating to the lips or to any lip-shaped structure.

la·cu'na   A small hollow or depression. In histology, the space in the matrix occupied by a cartilage cell or by the body of a bone cell.

la·mel'la   A thin sheetlike layer, such as the lamella of a bone.

lam'i·na pro'pri·a   A connective tissue layer. Also called tunica propria.

leu'ko·cyte   One of the colorless, more or less ameboid cells of the blood, having a nucleus and cytoplasm.

Leydig, cells of The interstitital cells of the testis.

Lieber·kühn, crypts of Simple straight tubular glands of the intestinal mucous membrane; slits from the base of the duodenal villi that extend into the mucosa as far as the muscularis mucosae. Excretory ducts of Brunner's glands usually open into these crypts. Also called intestinal glands, mucous crypts.

lobe One of the subdivisions of an organ or other part of the body, bounded by fissures, connective tissue, septa, or other structural markings.

lob'ule A small lobe.

lon″gi·tu'di·nal sec'tion A section cut lengthwise in the direction of the long axis of a structure.

lu'men The cavity or passageway of a tubular organ, as the lumen of the digestive or respiratory tract.

lu'nu·la The white semilunar area of a nail near the root.

lymph The fluid contained in the lymphatic vessels, composed of plasma and white blood cells.

lym'pho·cyte A cell formed primarily in lymphoid tissue in many parts of the body.

ly'so·somes Lysosomes provide hydrolytic enzymes for digestion of some of the materials taken into the cells.

mac'ro·phage A phagocytic cell belonging to the reticuloendothelial system.

Martinotti's cells Nerve cells in the cerebral cortex with axons running toward the surface and ramifying horizontally.

ma'trix The intercellular substances of a tissue, as of cartilage.

me·a'tus An opening or passage.

me″di·as·ti'num A partition separating adjacent parts.

me·dul'la The central part of certain organs as distinguished from the cortex.

Meis'sner, cor'pus·cles of Ovoid corpuscles connected with one or more myelinated nerve fibers which lose their sheaths as they enter a surrounding capsule, make several spiral turns, and break up into a complex network of branches.

mem'brane A limiting protoplasmic surface.

mem'brane bone A bone formed by, or within, a connective tissue, without a cartilaginous model.

Mer'kel's disks Tactile nerve endings.

mer'o·crine gland A gland in which the act of secretion leaves the cell intact throughout the cyclic process of formation and discharge.

mes'en·chyme A loose embryonic connective tissue derived chiefly from mesoderm, although some of its cells may have an ectodermal or entodermal origin.

mes″·o·the′li·um   A simple squamous epithelium, lining the serous cavities (pleura, pericardium, peritoneum).

mi·crog′li·a   Small neuroglia cells of the central nervous system.

mi′cron   One one-thousandth part of a millimeter.

mi″·cro·vil′li   Numerous folds in the luminal surface of the cell.

mil′li·me″ter   One one-thousandth part of a meter.

mil″·li·mi′cron   One one-thousandth part of a micron.

mit″·o·chon′dri·a   Small cytoplasmic structures. Electron microscopy shows mitochondria as membranous structures consisting of an outer limiting membrane and an inner corrugated membrane with cristae continuous with the inner limiting membrane. They are the sites of respiratory enzymes of the cell.

mon′o·cyte   A large mononuclear leukocyte with a more or less deeply indented nucleus, slate-gray cytoplasm, and fine, usually azurophilic granulation.

mu·co′sa   Mucous membrane consisting of an epithelium with some subepithelial connective tissue that lines cavities that communicate with the exterior. In some cases, as in the digestive tract, the mucosa includes the muscularis mucosae.

mu′cous   Pertaining to mucus.

mu′cus   A lubricating substance containing antibacterial enzymes and composed of water, mucin, a mucoprotein or carbohydrate-protein complex.

mul″·ti·cel′lu·lar   Consisting of many cells.

mul″·ti·po′lar   Having more than one pole, as multipolar nerve cells; those having more than one process.

mus″·cu·lar′is mu·co′sae   The single or double thin layer of smooth muscle in the deep portion of some mucous membranes, as in most of the digestive tube.

my′e·lin   The white fatty substance forming a sheath of some nerves, also called white substance of Schwann. By electron microscopy, the myelin sheath represents concentric layers of plasma membrane formed as a result of the Schwann cells wrapping themselves around the axis cylinder again and again.

my″·en·ter′ic   Relating to the muscular coat of the intestine.

my″·o·car′di·um   The muscular tissue of the heart.

my″·o·ep″·i·the′li·al cells   Smooth muscle cells in certain glands that develop from the same epithelium as the glandular elements.

my″·o·fi′bril   One of numerous longitudinal fibrils contained within the protoplasm of the muscle cell or fiber.

na″·so·phar′ynx   The space behind the posterior nares and above a horizontal plane through the lower margin of the palate.

neu″ri·lem′ma   The cellular sheath enclosing a nerve fiber. Also called neurolemma.

neu·rog′li·a   A general term for the fibrous and cellular, nonnervous, supporting elements of the nervous system chiefly derived from ectoderm.

neu′ron, neu′rone   The nerve cell composed of the cell body with its processes.

neu′tro·phil   Any histologic element readily stainable with neutral dyes. The polymorphonuclear leukocyte of the blood which contains neutrophil granules in its cytoplasm.

nis′sl bod′ies   Chromophil substance of nerve cells; consists of ribonucleoprotein.

node of Ran″vi·er′   A node in a myelinated nerve produced by a local constriction in the myelin sheath at an interval of about 50 to 1,000 microns.

nu′cle·ar mem′brane   Thin film separating the nucleus from the surrounding cytoplasm. Under the electron microscope the nuclear membrane consists of a pair of membranes with cisterna between them.

nu·cle′o·lus   A small spherical body within the cell nucleus.

nu′cle·o·plasm   The protoplasm of the nucleus.

nu′cle·us   The denser portion of the protoplasm of a cell, usually ovoid or globular in shape. It contains the hereditary material (DNA) and controls synthesis of protein by the cell.

o·don′to·blast   A dentin-forming cell.

ol″i·go·den′dro·cyte   Small supporting cells of the nervous system, located about the nerve cells, between nerve fibers and along blood vessels, and characterized by spheroidal or ovoid nuclei and fine cytoplasmic processes with secondary divisions.

op′ti·cal sec′tion   The field in sharp focus at any plane below the surface of a more or less transparent specimen when seen through the microscope.

or′gan   A group of cells or tissues that are associated in the body to perform one or more special functions.

or′gan of Cor′ti   A complex membranous structure in the cochlea; the organ of hearing.

or′gan sys′tem   The sum of the organs that serve for a general function.

or″gan·elle′   A specialized structure or part of a cell having a definite function to perform.

o″ro·phar′ynx   Situated below the level of the lower border of the soft palate and above the larynx, as distinguished from the nasopharynx and laryngeal pharynx.

os″si·fi·ca′tion   The formation of bone; the conversion of tissue into bone.

os′te·o·blast″   A bone-forming cell.

os′te·o·clast″ A large multinucleated cell associated with resorption of bone. The cell forms as the result of fusion of single-nucleated cells, and as a result forms with one or few nuclei. These cells are very rich in mitochondria and stand out in preparations stained for mitochondria.

os′te·o·cyte″ A bone cell.

os″te·o·gen′e·sis The development of bony tissue.

ox·yn′tic Secreting acid, formerly applied to the parietal cells of the stomach.

ox′y·phil Attracting acid dyes.

Pa·cin′i·an cor′pus·cle A large elliptical corpuscle made up of many concentric lamellas of connective tissue around a core containing the termination of a nerve fiber. It functions as a pressure receptor.

Pa′neth cells Large cells containing eosinophilic granules found at the blind extremity of the fundus of the intestinal glands (crypts of Lieberkühn).

pa·pil′la A small, nipplelike eminence.

par″a·u·re′thral Beside the urethra.

pa·ren′chy·ma The specific tissue component of an organ, such as hepatic cells in the liver.

pa·ri′e·tal Relating to the wall of any cavity.

pa·rot′id Situated near the ear, as the parotid gland.

pars con″vo·lu′ta The convoluted part or labyrinth of the kidney.

per″i·chon′dri·um A dense connective tissue sheath that covers the surface of cartilage.

per′i·cyte A special cell sometimes seen around a capillary or capillary arteriole with dendritic processes about the vessel and exhibiting contractile properties, similar to Rouget cells.

per″i·neu′ri·um The connective tissue sheath investing a primary bundle of nerve fibers.

per″i·o·don′tal Surrounding a tooth, as the periodontal membrane.

per″i·os′te·um The outer modified connective tissue covering of a bone.

pe·riph′er·y The outer part or surface; the part of the body away from the center.

per″me·a·bil′i·ty Property of membranes which permits transit of molecules and ions.

Pey′er's patch′es Aggregations of lymph nodules in the mucous membrane of the ileum opposite the mesenteric attachment.

phag′o·cyte A cell having the property of engulfing and digesting foreign or other particles or cells harmful to the body.

phos′pha·tase A type of enzyme that catalyzes the hydrolysis of esters of phosphoric acid. Numerous phosphatases are known to exist and they play an important role in carbohydrate metabolism, in nucleotide metabolism, in phospholipid metabolism, and in bone formation.

phos″pho·lip′id   A type of lipid compound which is an ester of phosphoric acid and contains, in addition, one or two molecules of fatty acid, an alcohol, and a nitrogenous base.

plas′ma mem′brane   Cell membrane.

plas″ma·lem′ma   Plasma membrane; cell membrane.

pli′ca   A bend or fold.

pli′cae cir″cu·lar′es   The shelflike folds of the mucous membrane of the small intestine.

pol″y·chro″ma·to·phil′ic   Referring to the ability of tissue to take stains of several kinds.

po·lyg′o·nal   Having many angles.

pol″y·mor″pho·nu′cle·ar   Having a nucleus in several forms.

pro·ges′ter·one   The hormone found in the corpus luteum.

pro·grav′id   Referring to the lutein phase of the endometrium.

pro′to·plasm   The essential substance of all living plant and animal cells.

pseu″do·strat′i·fied ep″i·the′li·um   Generally, a simple columnar epithelium in which cells of varying height all touch the basement membrane, but only a few reach the surface. The nuclei are at different levels.

Pur·kin′je fibers   The modified cardiac muscle fibers of the conduction system of the heart.

ra′di·al sec′tion   A section, the parts of which radiate in all directions from a given center.

Ran″vi·er′, node of   A node in a myelinated nerve produced by a local constriction in the myelin sheath at an interval of about 50 to 1,000 microns.

re′nal cor′pus·cle   Clustered capillaries (glomerulus) surrounded by the expanded portion of the uriniferous tubule (Bowman's capsule) of the kidney.

re′te tes′tis   The network of anastomosing tubules in the mediastinum testis.

re·tic′u·lar   Resembling a net; formed by a network, as a reticular tissue.

re·tic″u·lo·en″do·the′li·al sys′tem   A group of different kinds of cells that have one physiological trait in common, namely, that all are phagocytic. Also called macrophage system.

rhom′bic   Having the form of an equilateral four-sided figure with opposite sides parallel and with angles, not right angles.

ri″bo·nu·cle′ic ac′id (RNA)   Genetic material in chromatin.

ri″bo·nu′cle·o·pro′te·in (RNP)   Dense granules along the outer surface of membranes of the ergastoplasm. The ribonucleoprotein fraction of the cell is considered the site of protein synthesis.

ri′bo·somes (ribonucleoprotein, RNP)   The chromidial substance; the cytoplasm of cells engaged in protein synthesis.

RNA   Ribonucleic acid. Genetic material in chromatin.

RNP   Ribonucleoprotein. Dense granules along the outer surface of mem-

branes of the ergastoplasm. The ribonucleoprotein fraction of the cell
is considered the site of protein synthesis.

Rou"get' cells   Similar to pericytes.

rou·leau'   A roll of red blood cells resembling a roll of coins.

ru'ga   A fold, wrinkle, elevation, or ridge.

sar"co·lem'ma   A delicate extracellular membrane surrounding striated
or skeletal muscle cells or fibers.

sar'co·mere   One of the segments into which a muscle fibril appears to
be divided by Z disks.

sar'co·plasm   The fluid protoplasmic substance of skeletal muscle cells.

Schmidt·Lan'ter·mann clefts   One of the oblique partitions interrupting
the myelin sheaths of each segment of a nerve fiber.

Schwann, sheath of   Neurilemma of a nerve fiber.

se·ba'ceous gland   One that secretes sebum, a fatty substance.

se·cre'to·ry duct   A smaller duct that is contributory to a gland's excretory ducts.

sep'tum   The wall or partition of connective tissue dividing an organ
or structure into two or more parts.

se"ro·mu'cous   Having the nature of or containing both serum and
mucus.

se·ro'sa   A serous membrane composed of mesothelium and subjacent
connective tissue, lining the pericardial, pleural, and peritoneal cavities
and covering their contents.

se'rous   Pertaining to, producing, or resembling serum.

Ser·to'li, cells of   Sustentacular cells of the seminiferous tubules.

se'rum   The fluid part of the blood and lymph remaining after coagula-
tion.

si'nus·oid   One of the relatively large spaces or tubes constituting part
of the venous circulatory system in the suprarenal gland, liver, and other
viscera.

Ske'ne's glands   Tubular mucous glands in the female urethra opening
just within the urinary meatus.

sphinc'ter   A ringlike muscle surrounding and closing an orifice.

squa'mous   Scalelike.

stel'late   Star-shaped.

ster"e·o·cil'i·um   A nonmotile cilium.

strat'i·fied   Arranged in layers, one above another.

stri'a·ted   Striped.

stro'ma   The connective tissue component of an organ.

sub'cu·ta'ne·ous   Beneath the skin.

sub·lin'gual   Lying beneath the tongue.

sub·max'il·lar"y   Lying beneath the lower maxilla or mandible.

sus″ten·tac′u·lar Supportive.

sus″ten·tac′u·lar cells Tall cells, irregular in outline, which extend from the basement membrane to the lumen. They support the germinal cells.

syn·cyt′i·um Protoplasm continued from one cell to another by uniting protoplasmic processes.

tac′tile Pertaining to the sense of touch.

tae′ni·ae co′li The three thick bands of the outer longitudinal muscle layer. In a given section, the longitudinal muscle layer may be thick or thin, depending on the presence of or absence of the taeniae coli.

ter′mi·nal bars The dense line that closes the intercellular spaces in various kinds of epithelia. It represents a modification of the cell surface and is related in structure to desmosomes (intercellular bridges) and intercalated disks of cardiac muscle.

the′ca fol′lic″u·li The capsule of a growing or mature ovarian follicle consisting of an inner vascular cellular layer and an outer fibrous layer.

throm′bo·cyte Blood platelet. Important in the clotting of blood.

throm″bo·plas′tid Blood platelet. Important in the clotting of blood.

tis′sue A group of cells of similar structure with intercellular substances that perform a specialized function.

tis′sue flu′id Extracellular fluid that is the environment of the body cells.

tra·bec′u·la A prolongation of a fibrous membrane forming septa or partitions.

trun′cat·ed Shortened in height.

tu′bu·li rec′ti Straight tubules.

tu″bu·lo·al·ve′o·lar Consisting of a system of branching tubules which terminate in alveoli, as in the salivary glands.

tu′ni·ca ad″ven·ti′ti·a The outer connective tissue coat of an organ where it is not covered by a serous membrane.

tu′ni·ca al″bu·gin′e·a tes′tis A layer of white fibrous tissue investing the testis. The outer layer consists of densely compacted collagenous and elastic fibers.

tu′ni·ca fi·bro′sa The sclera.

tu′ni·ca in′ti·ma The inner coat of a blood or lymph vessel.

tu′ni·ca me′di·a The middle coat of a blood or lymph vessel.

tu′ni·ca se·ro′sa The mesothelium and underlying connective tissue forming the visceral and parietal pericardium, pleura, peritoneum, and tunica vaginalis propria testis.

tu′ni·ca vas″cu·lo′sa tes′tis A layer of loose connective tissue containing many blood vessels on the inner surface of the tunica albuginea testis.

ver′ti·cal sec′tion A section cut perpendicularly to the surface of a structure.

Volk′mann's canals   Small canals found in bone which transmit blood vessels.

zo′na pel·lu′cid·a   The thick solid elastic envelope of the ovum.

zy″mo·gen′ic   Causing fermentation. Zymogen cells are the inactive precursors of an enzyme, which, on reaction with the appropriate kinase or other chemical agent, liberates the enzyme in active form.

SELECTED REFERENCES

Andrews, W.: *Textbook of Comparative Histology,* Oxford University Press, Fair Lawn, N.J., 1959.

Arey, L. B.: *Developmental Anatomy,* W. B. Saunders Company, Philadelphia, 1965.

Arey, L. B.: *Human Histology,* 2d ed., W. B. Saunders Company, Philadelphia, 1963.

Baker, J. R.: *Principles of Biological Microtechnique,* John Wiley & Sons, New York, 1958.

Bargmann, W.: *Histologie und mikroskopische Anatomie des Menschen,* Georg Thieme Verlag, Stuttgart, 1951.

Bloom, W., and D. W. Fawcett: *A Textbook of Histology,* 8th ed., W. B. Saunders Co., Philadelphia, 1964.

Clark, W. E. LeGros: *The Tissues of the Body,* Oxford University Press, Fair Lawn, N.J., 1958.

Conn, H. J.: *Biological Stains,* 6th ed., Biotech Publications, Geneva, N.Y., 1953.

Copenhaver, W. M., and D. D. Johnson: *Bailey's Textbook of Histology,* 15th ed., The Williams & Wilkins Company, Baltimore, 1964.

Cowdry, E. V.: *A Textbook of Histology: Functional Significance of Cells and Intercellular Substances,* 4th ed., Lea & Febiger, Philadelphia, 1950.

De Robertis, E. D. P., W. W. Nowinski, and F. A. Saez: *General Cytology,* 3d ed., W. B. Saunders Company, Philadelphia, 1960.

Di Fiore, M. S. H.: *Atlas of Human Histology,* 2d ed., Lea & Febiger, Philadelphia, 1963.

Freeman, J. A.: *Cellular Fine Structure: An Introductory Student Text and Atlas,* McGraw-Hill Book Company, New York, 1964.

Gillison, M.: *Histology of Body Tissue,* The Williams & Wilkins Company, Baltimore, 1950.

Gomori, G.: *Microscopic Histochemistry,* The University of Chicago Press, Chicago, 1953.

Gray, E.: *Electron Microscopy in Anatomy,* The Williams & Wilkins Company, Baltimore, 1961.

Greep, R. O. (ed.): *Histology,* 2d ed., McGraw-Hill Book Company, New York, 1966.

Ham, A. W.: *Histology,* 3d ed., J. B. Lippincott Company, Philadelphia, 1957.

Hoskins, M. M., and G. Bevelander: *Essentials of Histology,* 3d ed., The C. V. Mosby Company, St. Louis, 1956.

Jordan, H. E.: *A Textbook of Histology,* 9th ed., Appleton-Century-Crofts, Inc., New York, 1952.

Porter, K. R., and M. A. Bonneville: *An Introduction to the Fine Structure of Cells and Tissues,* 2d ed., Lea & Febiger, Philadelphia, 1964.

Rhodin, J. A. G.: *An Atlas of Ultrastructure,* W. B. Saunders Company, Philadelphia, 1963.

Stöhr, Philipp: *Lehrbuch der Histologie und der mikroskopischen Anatomie des Menschen,* Springer-Verlag OHG, Berlin, 1951.

Trautmann, A., and J. Fiebiger: *Fundamentals of the Histology of Domestic Animals,* 2d ed., Comstock Publishing Associates, a division of Cornell University Press, Ithaca, N.Y., 1957.

Von Herrath, E., and S. Abramow: *Atlas der normalen Histologie und mikroskopischen Anatomie des Menschen,* Georg Thieme Verlag, Stuttgart, 1950.

Werner, H. J.: *Synopsis of Histology,* 2d ed., McGraw-Hill Book Company, New York, 1967.

Windle, W. F.: *Textbook of Histology,* 3d ed., McGraw-Hill Book Company, New York, 1960.

INDEX

Acidophils, 62
Adipose tissue, 44
Adrenal glands, 200
Adventitia, 164
Afferent receptors, 78
Agranulocytes, 60
Albuginea, 170
Alveolus, lungs, 158
  tooth, 128
Amitosis, 18
Ampulla, of ductus deferens, 172
  of ear, 214
  of Vater, 138
Anal canal, 142
Appendages of skin, 112
Appendix, 140
Areola, 190
Areolar connective tissue, 38
Argentaffine cells, 138
Arteries, 86
  elastic, 88
  muscular type, 86
Arterioles, 86
Arteriovenous anastomoses, 88
Articular cartilage, 46
Astrocytes, 80
Atria of heart, 94
Atrioventricular bundle of His, 94
Auditory tube, 212
Auricle of ear, 212
Axoplasm, 72

Basophils, 62, 194
Beta cells, 194
Bile duct, 152
  common, 152
Bipolar cell, 74
Bladder, urinary, 164
    mucosa of, 164
    muscularis of, 164
    serosa of, 166
Blood, 58
  plasma, 62
  platelets, 62, 64
  red corpuscles, 58

Blood, summary of formed elements in
  blood, 64
  white corpuscles, 58
Bone, 50
  cancellous, 50
  compact, 50
  development of, 50
  endochondral ossification of, 52
  intracartilaginous ossification of, 52
  intramembranous ossification of, 50
  osteogenesis, 50
  spongy, 50
Bowman's membrane, 204
Bronchi, 156
Bronchioles, 158
Brunner's glands, 138
Brush border, cell, 16
Buccal glands, 150
Bulbourethral glands, 174

Cancellous bone, 50
Capillaries, 86, 98
Cardiac of stomach, 134
Cardiac glands, 132
Cardiac muscle, 68, 70, 78
Cartilage, 44
  articular, 46
  diagram of, 40
  distribution of, 223
  elastic, 46
  gristle, 44
  hyaline, 46
  precartilage, 44
  white fibrocartilage, 46
Cecum, 140
Cell, 10
  albuminous, 34
  alpha, 194
  argentaffine, 138
  beta, 194
  bipolar, 74
  centroacinous, 150
  chief, 134, 198
  chromophil, 194
  chromophobe, 194

Cell, division of, 18
  amitosis, direct, 18
  mitosis, indirect, 20
  goblet, 32, 138
  gustatory, 220
  interstitial, 170, of testis, 200
  of Leydig, 170
  monopolar, 72
  mucous, 32
  multipolar, 74
  nerve, 72
  Paneth, 138
  prismatic, 24
  Purkinje, 82
  serous, 34
  sustentacular, 170, 218, 228
  unipolar, 72
Cell structure, 10
  brush border, 16
  centrosome, 10, 12
  cilia, 16
  cristae, 10
  cytoplasm, 10
    inclusions, 12, 16
  desmosome, 16
  diplosome, 10
  endoplasmic reticulum, 12, 14
    agranular, 12, 14
    granular, 12
    rough, 12
    smooth, 12, 14
  ergastoplasm, 12, 14
  flagella, 16
  intercellular bridges, 18, 22
  interdigitation, 18
  meiosis, 20
    diploid, 20
    haploid, 20
  membrane, 10, 12
  microvilli, 16
  nucleus, 18
  organelles, 10, 11
  organoids, 10
  plasma membrane, 12, 16
  plasmalemma, 12, 16
  ribonucleoprotein, 12, 14
  ribosomes, 14
  RNP, 14
  stereocilia, 16
  sterols, 14
  striated border, 16
  terminal bars, 16
Cementocytes, 128
Cementum, 128
Centriole, cell, 10
Centroacinous cells, 150
Centrosome, cell, 10
Cerebellum, 82

Cerebrum, 84
  ganglionic layer, 84
  inner granular, 84
  molecular layer, 82
  multiform layer, 84
  outer granular, 82
  plexiform layer, 82
  pyramidal cell layer, 82
  white matter, 84
  zonal layer, 82
Cervix, 186
Chordae tendineae, 94
Choroid, 206
Chromophil substance, 72
Chromosomes, 18
Cilia, 16
Ciliary body, 206
Circulatory system, 86
  arteries, 86, 88
  arterioles, 86
  arteriovenous anastomoses, 88
  capillaries, 86
  coccygeal body, 88
  glomus coccygeum, 88
  heart, 94
  lymphatic vessels, 92, 100
  sinusoids, 92, 100
  summary of histology of, 98, 100
  tunica adventitia, 86, 88, 90, 92
  tunica intima, 86, 88, 90
  tunica media, 86, 90
  valves, 92, 96
  vasa vasorum, 92
  veins, 90, 92
Clasmatocytes, 54
Classification, simple epithelial tissues,
    22, 28
  stratified epithelial tissues, 24
Coccygeal body, 88
Cochlea, 214
Cohnheim's fields, 68
Collagenous fibers, 38
Colon, 140
Compact bone, 50
Connective tissue, 36
  adipose, 44
  adult, 38
  areolar, 38
  bone, 50
    development of, 50
  cartilage, 46
  dense, 42
  diagram of types, 40, 48
  elastic, 44
  embryonic, 36
  gristle, 44
  loose, 38
  mesenchyme, 36

Connective tissue, mucous, 38
  collagenous fibers, 38
  pigmented, 44
  reticular, 42
  yellow elastic, 44
Convoluted tubules, 170
Corium, 114
Cornea, 204
Corneal stroma, 204
Corpus luteum of ovary, 182
Corpuscles, 58
  agranulocytes, 60
  basophils, 62
  crenated, 58
  eosinophils, 62
  erythrocytes, 58
  erythroplastid, 58
  granulocytes, 60
  leukocytes, 58
    polymorphonuclear, 60
  lymphocytes, 60
  of Meissner, touch, 78
  Merkel's, 78
  monocytes, 60
  neutrophils, 60
  Pacinian, 78
  red, 58
  rouleaux, 58
  tactile, 78
  of Vater-Pacini, 78
  white, 58
Cortex of kidney, 162
Cowper's gland, 174
Crenated corpuscles, 58
Cristae, 10
Cuboidal epithelium, 24, 28, 30
Cytoplasm of nerve cells, 72
Cytoplasmic inclusions, 16

Dense connective tissue, 42
Dental pulp, 128
Dentin, 126
Dentinal canals, 128
Derma, 114
Dermis, 114
Descemet's membrane, 204
Desmosomes, 16
Diagrams, connective tissue, 40, 48
  epithelial, 30, 32
  how to interpret sections, 2–5
Digestive system, 122
  esophagus, 130
  gastroesophageal junction, 132
  glands, 148
  intestine, large, 140
    small, 126
  lips, 122

Digestive system, mouth, 124
  oral cavity, 124
  palate, 128
  pharynx, 130
  stomach, 134
  summary of, 144–147
  teeth, 124
  tongue, 124
Diplosome, 10
Distribution of cartilage, 223
Ductless glands, 194
Ductuli efferentes, 172
Ductus deferens, 172
Ductus epididymis, 172
Duodenum, 138

Ear, 212
  external, 212
  inner, 214
  middle, 212
Eardrum, 212
Ejaculatory ducts, 174
Elastic cartilage, 46
Elastic tissue, 44
Electron microscope, 8, 9, 12, 14, 72
Embryonic connective tissue, 36
  mesenchyme, 36
  mucous, 38
Enamel, teeth, 126
Encapsulated nerve endings, 78
Endocardium, 94
Endochondral ossification, 52
Endocrine system, 194
  adrenal glands, 200
  corpus luteum of ovary, 182
  epiphysis, 202
  hypophysis, 194
  interstitial cells, testis, 170
  islets of Langerhans, 200
  pancreatic islands, 200
  parathyroid, 198
  pineal body, 202
  pituitary gland, 194
  suprarenal glands, 200
  thymus, 104, 202
  thyroid, 196
Endometrium, 184
Endoneurium, 74
Endoplasmic reticulum, 12, 14
  agranular, 14
  granular, 12
  rough, 12
  smooth, 14
Eosinophils, 62
Ependyma, 82
Epicardium, 94
Epidermis, 112

Epidermis, granular layer, 112
  Malpighian layer, 112
  stratum corneum, 114
  stratum germinativum, 112
  stratum granulosum, 112
  stratum lucidum, 114
Epineurium, 74
Epiphysis, 202
Episcleral tissue, 204
Epithelial tissues, 22–34
  ciliated and non-ciliated, 22, 24, 28
  classification, 22, 28
    simple, 22, 28
      columnar, 24, 28, 30, 32
      cuboidal, 24, 28, 30, 32
      pseudostratified, 24, 28, 30, 32
      squamous, 22, 28, 30, 32
    stratified, 24, 29, 30
      columnar, 29, 30, 32
      squamous, 26, 29, 30, 32
      transitional, 26, 29, 30, 32
  diagrams, types of epithelial tissues,
    30, 32
  glandular, 32
    multicellular, 32
    unicellular, 32
  neuroepithelia, 34
  pigmented, 34
  summary of, 32
Eponychium, 120
Ergastoplasm, 12, 14
Erythrocytes, 58, 64
Erythroplastids, 58
Esophageal glands, 132
Esophagus, 130
Eustachian tube, 212
External auditory meatus, 210
Eye, 204
  choroid, 206
  ciliary body, 206
  cornea, 204
  eyelids, 210
  iris, 206
  lacrimal glands, 210
  lens, 208
  optic nerve, 210
  retina, 208
  sclera, 204
  tunica fibrosa, 204
  vitreous body, 210
Eyelids, 210

Fallopian tube, 182
Fibrils (fibrillae), 14
Flagella, 16
Follicular structure, 116
Foreskin, 176

Fundus of stomach, 134

Gallbladder, 152
Ganglia, 76
  autonomic, 76
  cerebrospinal, 76
Gastroesophageal junction, 132
Glands, of digestive system, 148
  Brunner's, 138
  buccal, 150
  cardiac, 134
  duodenal, 138
  gallbladder, 152
  liver, 150
  pancreas, 150
  salivary, 148
    buccal, 150
    labial, 150
    lingual, 150
    oral, 150
    palatine, 150
    parotid, 148
    sublingual, 148
    submaxillary, 148
  of endocrine system, 194
    adrenal, 200
    corpus luteum, 200
    epiphysis, 202
    hypophysis, 194
    interstitial cells of testis, 200
    Langerhans, islets of, 200
    pancreatic islands, 200
    parathyroid, 198
    pineal body, 202
    pituitary, 194
    suprarenal, 200
    thymus, 202
    thyroid, 196
  of reproductive system, 174
    female, mammary gland, 188
    male, bulbourethral, 174
      Cowper's, 174
  of skin, 118
    sebaceous, 118
    sweat, 118
  of urinary system, 166
    paraurethral, 166
Glandular epithelia, 32
  multicellular glands, 32
  unicellular glands. 32
Glassy membrane, 182, 206
Glia, 80
Glisson, islands of, 152
Globules, 16
Glomus coccygeum, 88
Glossary, 225
Goblet cells, 138

Golgi apparatus, 14
 organs of, 80
Graafian follicle, 180
Granular layer, 112
 inner, 82
Granulocytes, 60
Gristle, 44
Gustatory cells, 220
Gustatory organ, 220
 taste buds, 220

Hair, 116
Heart, 94
 atria, 94
 atrioventricular bundle of His, 94
 chordae tendineae, 94
 endocardium, 94
 epicardium, 94
 impulse conducting system, 94
 myocardium, 94
 valves, 94
 ventricles, 94
Hemal nodes, 102
Hemolymph nodes, 102
Henle's loop, 162
Histocytes, 54
Hyaline cartilage, 46
Hypodermis, 114
Hyponychium, 120
Hypophysis, 194

Identification methods of tissues and organs, 6
 microscopic, 7
 recognition of elements, 6, 8
 superficial recognition, 7
Ileum, 138
Inner ear, 214
Integument, 112
Intercalated disk, 68
Intercellular bridges, 18, 22
Interdigitation, 18
Interphase cell, 20
Interpretation of section, 1–5
Interstitial cells of testis, 170
Intervertebral disk, 46
Intestinal glands, 136, 138, 140
Intestines, 136
 glands, 138
 large, 140
 anal canal, 142
 cecum, 140
 colon, 140
 rectum, 142
 vermiform appendix, 140
 small, 138

Intestines, small, mucosa, 136
 muscularis, 136
 serosa, 136
 specific regions, 138
 duodenum, 138
 ileum, 138
 jejunum, 138
 submucosa, 136
 wall, 136
Intracartilaginous ossification, 52
Intramembranous ossification, 52
Involuntary muscle, 66
Iris, 206
Ischemic phase, 186
Islets of Langerhans, 200

Jejunum, 138

Kidney, 162
Kupffer cells, 54

Labial gland, 150
Labyrinth, 214
Lacrimal glands, 210
Lamellar corpuscles, 78
Lamina fusca, 204
Lamina propria, 126, 164, 218
Lamina vasculosa, 206
Langerhans, islets of, 200
Larynx, 154
Lens, 208
Leukocytes, 58, 64
Leydig, cells of, 170
Lieberkühn, crypts of, 138
 glands of, 138
Lingual glands, 150
Lingual tonsil, 106
Lips, 122
Littré, glands of, 166
Liver, 150
Loose connective tissue, 38
Lung, 158
Lunula, 120
Lymph, 58, 62
Lymph nodes, 102
Lymphatic organs, 102
 hemal nodes, 102
 lymph nodes, 102
 spleen, 104
 summary of lymphatic organs, 110
 thymus, 104
 tonsil, 104
Lymphatic vessels, 92
Lymphocytes, 60
Lysosomes, 14

Macrophage system, 54
Macrophages, 54
Malpighian layer, 112
Mammary gland, 188
  active, 190
  involution, 190
  resting, 188
  retrogressive, 190
Matrix, nail, 120
Medulla, kidney, 162
Medullated nerve fibers, 74
Meiosis, 20
  diploid, 20
  haploid, 20
Meissner, touch corpuscle of, 78
Meissner's nerve plexus, 134, 140
Merkel's corpuscles, 78
Merkel's disks, 78
Mesenchyme, 36
Microglia, 56, 80
Microvilli, 16
Middle ear, 212
Mitochondria, 10
Mitosis, 20
  anaphase, 20
  metaphase, 20
  prophase, 20
  telophase, 20
Monocytes, 60
Monopolar cell, 72
Motor nerve endings, 76
Mouth, 124
  mucosa, 124
  mucous membrane, 124
  submucosa, 124
Mucous tissue, 38
Multicellular glands, 32
Muscle spindles, 80
Muscle tendon spindles, 80
Muscular coat of ureter, 164
Muscular tissues, 66
  cardiac, 68, 70
  nonstriated, 66
  skeletal, 68, 70
  smooth, 66, 70
  striated, 68
Muscularis, externa, 130
Myelinated nerve fibers, 74
Myenteric plexus, 140
Myocardium, 94
Myofibrils, 68
Myometrium, 186

Nails, 120
  bed, 120
  body, 120
  eponychium, 120

Nails, hyponychium, 120
  lunula, 120
  matrix, 120
  plate, 120
  root, 120
  wall, 120
Nasal cavity, 154
Nasopharynx, 154
Nervi vasorum, 88
Nervous tissue, 72
  autonomic ganglia, 76
  cells, nerve, 72
  cerebellum, 82
  cerebrospinal ganglia, 76
  cerebrum, 82
  motor nerve endings, 76
  myelinated nerve fibers, 74
  neuroglia, 80
  neurons, 72
  sensory nerve endings, 78
  spinal cord, 82
  unmyelinated nerve fibers, 74
Neurilemma, 74
Neuroepithelia, 34
Neurofibrils, 72
Neuroglia, 80
Neurolemma, 74
Neuromuscular bundles, 80
Neurons, 72
Neutrophils, 60
Nipple, 190
Nissl bodies, 72
Nonencapsulated endings, 78
Nonmedullated nerve fibers, 76
Nonstriated muscle, 66
Nucleolus, 18
Nucleus, 18

Odontoblasts, 128
Olfactory epithelium, 218
Olfactory organ, 218
Oligodendrocytes, 80
Oligodendroglia, 80
Oocyte, 180
Optic nerve, 210
Oral cavity, 124
Oral gland, 150
Organ of Corti, 216
Organelles, 10, 11
Organoids, 10
Organs and tissues that may be confused,
  221
Ossification, intracartilaginous, 52
  intramembranous, 52
Osteogenesis, 50
Ovary, 180

Oviduct, 182

Pacinian corpuscles, 78
Palate, 128
Palatine gland, 150
Palatine tonsil, 106
Pancreas, 150
Pancreatic islands, 200
Paneth cells, 138
Papillae, tongue, 124
Papillary muscle, heart, 94
Parathyroid, 198
Paraurethral glands, 166
Parotid, 148
Pars cavernosum, 166
Pars distalis, 194
Pars intermedia, 196
Pars membranacea, 166
Pars nervosa, 196
Pars prostatica, 166
Pars tuberalis, 196
Pelvis of kidney, 164
Penis, 176
Perikaryon, 72
Perimetrium, 186
Perineurium, 74
Periodontal membrane, 128
Peyer's patches, 138
Pharyngeal tonsil, 106
Pharynx, 130, 154
Phosphatase activity, 14
Phospholipid, 14
Pigmentation, 114
Pigmented epithelium, 34
Pigmented tissue, 44
Pineal body, 202
Pinna, 212
Pituitary gland, 194
Placenta, 186
Plasma, 62
  membrane, 16
Plasmalemma, 16
Platelets, blood, 62, 64
Polymorphonuclear leukocytes, 60
Portal canal, 152
Precartilage, 44
Prepuce, 176
Prostate gland, 174
Protein synthesis, 14
Pseudostratified epithelium, 24, 28, 30, 32
Pulp tissue, 128
Purkinje's cells, 82
  fibers, 96
Pylorus of stomach, 136
Pyramidal layer, 82

Rectum, 142
References, 241
Reproductive system, 170
  female, 180
    cervix, 186
    corpus luteum, 182
    Fallopian tube, 182
    mammary gland, 188
    ovary, 180
    oviduct, 182
    placenta, 186
    summary, 192
    uterine tube, 182
    uterus, 184
    vagina, 188
  male, 170
    bulbourethral glands, 174
    ductuli efferentes, 172
    ductus deferens, 172
    ejaculatory ducts, 174
    ductus epididymis, 172
    penis, 176
    prostate gland, 174
    seminal vesicles, 174
    summary, 178, 179
    testis, 170
Respiratory system, 154
  bronchi, 156
  bronchioles, 158
  larynx, 154
  lung, 158
  nasal cavity, 154
  nasopharynx, 154
  pharynx, 154
  summary, 160, 161
  trachea, 156
Rete testis, 172
Reticular cells, 56
  tissue, 42
Reticuloendothelial system, 54
  clasmatocytes, 54
  histocytes, 54
  Kupffer cells, 54
  macrophages, 54
  microglia, 56
  resting wandering cells, 54
  reticular cells, 56
Retina, 208
Ribonucleoprotein, 12, 14, 72
Ribosomes, 14
RNP, 14, 72
Root sheath, 116
Rouleaux, 58

Saccule, 214
Salivary glands, 148
Sarcolemma, 70

Sclera, 204
Scrotum, 114
Sebaceous glands, 118
Secretion granules, 16
Sections, interpretation of, 1–5
Semicircular canals, 214
Seminal vesicles, 174
Seminiferous epithelium, 170
  tubules, 170
Sensory nerve endings, 78
Seromucous glands, 34
Serous cells, 34
Sertoli cells, 170
Sheath of Schwann, 74
Simple epithelia, 22, 28
Sinusoids, 92
Skeletal muscle, 68, 70
Skin, 112
  dermis, 112
  epidermis, 112
  follicle, 116
  glands, 118
  hair, 116
  hypodermis, 114
  nails, 120
  pigmentation, 114
  of scrotum, 114
  subcutaneous tissue, 114
  tela subcutanea, 114
Smooth muscle, 66, 70
Spinal cord, 82
Spleen, 104
Spongy bone, 50
Squamous epithelium, 22, 26
Stereocilia, 16
Sterols, 14
Stomach, 132
  mucosa, 132
  regions of, 134
    cardiac, 134
    cardiac glands, 134
    fundus, 134
    pylorus, 136
  serosa, 134
  submucosa, 134
  submucous nerve plexus, 134
  wall, 132
Stratified epithelia, 24, 29, 30, 32
Stratum corneum, 114
Stratum germinativum, 112
Stratum granulosum, 112
Stratum lucidum, 114
Striated border, 16
  muscle, 68
Subcutaneous tissue, 114
Subcutis, 114
Sublingual gland, 148
Submandibular gland, 148

Submaxillary gland, 148
Summary, of blood, 64
  of circulatory system, 97–99
  of digestive system, 144–147
  of distribution of cartilage, 223
  of epithelial tissues, 32
  of lymphatic organs, 110
  of reproductive system, 178, 179, 192
    female, 192
    male, 178, 179
  of respiratory system, 160, 161
  of urinary system, 168, 169
Suprachoroid layer, 206
Suprarenal glands, 200
Sustentacular cells, taste organs, 220
  of testis, 170
Sweat glands, 118

Tactile corpuscles, 78
Taste buds, 220
Taste organs, 220
Tectorial membrane, 216
Teeth, 126
  cementum, 128
  dental pulp, 128
  dentin, 128
  dentinal canals, 128
  enamel, 126
  odontoblasts, 128
  periodontal membrane, 128
  pulp tissue, 128
  Tomes' dentinal fibrils, 128
Tela subcutania, 114
Terminal bars, 16
Testicle, 170
Testis, 170
Thrombocytes, 62
Thromboplastids, 62
Thymus, 104, 202
Thyroid, 196
Tissues and organs that may be con-
  fused, 221
Tomes' dentinal fibrils, 128
Tongue, 124
Tonsil, 106
  lingual, 106
  palatine, 106
  pharyngeal, 106
  tubal, 108
Touch corpuscle of Meissner, 78
Trachea, 156
Transitional epithelium, 26
Trinity, portal canal, 152
Tubal tonsil, 106
Tubules, distal convoluted, 162
  proximal convoluted, 162
Tubuli efferentes, 172

Tubuli recti, 170
Tunica adventitia, 90
Tunica fibrosa, 204
Tunica intima, 90
Tunica media, 90
Tunica propria, 124, 126
Tunica of testis, 170
Tympanic cavity, 212

Unicellular glands, 32
Unipolar cell, 72
Unmyelinated nerve fibers, 76
Ureter, 164
  adventitia, 164
  mucosa, 164
  muscularis, 164
Urethra, female, 166
  male, 166
Urinary system, 162
  bladder, 164
  kidney, 162
  summary of, 168, 169
  ureter, 164
  urethra, female, 166
    male, 166
    Littré, glands of, 166
Uterine tubes, 182
Uterus, 184
Utricle, 214

Vagina, 188
  adventitia, 188

Vagina, mucosa, 188
  muscularis, 188
  submucosa, 188
Valves, of heart, 94
  of large-sized veins, 92
Vas deferens, 172
Vasa vasorum, 92
Vasculosa, 170
Vater, ampulla of, 138
Vater-Pacini, corpuscles of, 78
Veins, 90
Ventricles, heart, 94
Vermiform appendix, 140
Vestibule, ear, 214
  nose, 154
Villi, 136, 138
Vitreous body, 210
Von Ebner, glands of, 150

Wandering cells, 54
White blood corpuscles, 58
White fibrocartilage, 46
White matter, 84

Yellow elastic tissue, 44

Zona fasciculata, 200
Zona glomerulosa, 200
Zona pellucida, 180
Zona reticularis, 200
Zymogenic cells, 134